HEALTH CARE POLICY IN THE UNITED STATES

edited by

JOHN G. BRUHN
PENNSYLVANIA STATE
UNIVERSITY-HARRISBURG

A GARLAND SERIES

Health Care Policy in the United States
John G. Bruhn, editor

DIRECTING HEALTH MESSAGES TOWARD AFRICAN AMERICANS

ATTITUDES TOWARD HEALTH CARE AND THE MASS MEDIA

JUDITH L. SYLVESTER

GARLAND PUBLISHING, INC.
A MEMBER OF THE TAYLOR & FRANCIS GROUP
NEW YORK & LONDON / 1998

Library of Congress Cataloging-in-Publication Data

Sylvester, Judith L.
　　Directing health messages toward African Americans :
attitudes toward health care and the mass media / Judith L.
Sylvester.
　　　　p.　　cm. — (Health care policy in the United States)
　　Includes bibliographical references and index.
　　ISBN 0-8153-3051-0 (alk. paper)
　　1. Afro-Americans—Health and hygiene. 2. Health attitudes—United States. 3. Afro-Americans—Attitudes. 4. Mass
media in health education—United States. 5. Afro-Americans and
mass media. 6. Medical care—United States—Marketing. I. Title.
II. Series: Health care policy in the United States (New York, N.Y.)
　　[DNLM: 1. Blacks—United States. 2. Health Services Accessi-
bility—United States. 3. Marketing of Health Services—methods.
4. Mass Media. WA 300 S985d 1997]
RA448.5.N4S95　1997
362.1'089'96073—dc21
DNLM/DLC
for Library of Congress　　　　　　　　　　　　　　97-42742

Dedication

For enduring from beginning to end, this book is dedicated to Jim, Jennifer, and Janelle Sylvester and to my parents, Nadine and Everett Smith, who have supported me in more ways than one.

Contents

List of Tables

Preface

Since the research for this book was completed in 1995, the Clinton Health Security Act of 1993 has vanished. The proposed comprehensive benefits that were to be guaranteed to every American never materialized. Pres. Clinton was never able to present an acceptable way to pay for the system, and Hillary Rodham Clinton, who spearheaded health care reform was relegated back to nearly invisible First Lady status.

After the Clinton plan failed, the health care issues flowed from a comprehensive river into specific-issue tributaries. When Congress takes up health care issues today, the debate is more likely to be about late-term abortion, Medicare reform, or tobacco and smoking regulations. Minority health care—especially preventive health care—has not become part of the national debate and likely will not do so during the 20th Century.

Congress passed a bill banning the so-called partial birth abortion procedure in 1996, but Clinton vetoed it because the bill would not allow the procedure to be used to protect a woman's health. Congress likely will make another attempt at passage before 1999.

Medicare, long considered a political sacred cow, has succumbed to the need for Congress and Pres. Clinton to balance the budget, eliminate waste and abuse and prevent Medicare from going broke in 2001. In response to an estimated $23 billion a year in waste and abuse, Congress has proposed raising the Medicare eligibility age from 65 to 67 in 2027, increasing premiums paid by upper-income seniors and strengthening Medicare's fraud and waste-busting powers. The plan also means that more elderly Americans will get their health care through health maintenance organizations and other managed care plans. Current estimates are that only about 13 % of Medicare beneficiaries are in managed care plans.[1]

What the impact of less Medicare and more managed care will be on the poorest people in American society has yet to be determined, but a recent government report found marketing abuses among Florida HMOs, such as sales staff targeting illiterate beneficiaries. Undoubtedly, minorities at the bottom of the socioeconomic scale are the most vulnerable if abuses in the system are not identified and prevented.

There are some positive signs in spite of the lack of national health care reform. More media attention has been focused on black health care issues, mostly the discrepancy of death rates from breast cancer between black and white women. Some articles in women's magazines now specifically mention the increased risk for black women when breast cancer and AIDS are discussed.

The national obsession with low fat diets and exercise has continued, although little information about diet and exercise is specifically targeted toward black Americans. (Where are the black Jane Fondas, Kathy Irelands and Bodies by Jake?) Still, a recent survey (conducted by the author) of college students in Baton Rouge, LA, does indicate that young blacks are less likely than their white counterparts to smoke. This is in spite of a great deal of advertising that has been aimed directly at them. Additionally, President Clinton has moved to regulate tobacco through the Food and Drug Administration and appears to have been successful in getting concessions from the tobacco industry that will restrict many forms of advertising aimed at young people.

Political correctness and research on black health care issues have clashed in a way that the research in this book perhaps could have predicted. *The Wall Street Journal*[2] reported on a controversy that arose when Memorial Sloan-Kettering Cancer Center conducted a survey as part of a larger breast-cancer research project. Dozens of black women in New York were asked questions that seemed to critics to be unrelated to health care. They were asked questions such as:

- Do you believe in voodoo?
- Do you trust root doctors?
- Do you feel most white people are racist?
- Do you eat chitlins once in a while?

To researchers who understand there can be differences between black and white cultures, these questions are acceptable, even necessary. However, critics found the survey to be racially insensitive. Marshall England, chairman of Harlem Hospital's community advisory board was quoted as saying:

> What do chitlins have to do with breast cancer? It is insulting, it is insensitive, it is provocative, and it is stereotyping.[3]

The Harlem chapter of the NAACP and the publisher of *The Amsterdam News* (an influential black newspaper) also condemned the survey, comparing the study to the notorious Tuskegee experiments that went on for forty years and allowed black men infected with syphilis to go untreated so that scientists could watch the progression of the disease.

According to the article, Sloan-Kettering's defense was:

> A predilection for chitlins (pig intestines, often deep-fried) would indicate a high-fat diet; a belief that most whites are racist could keep black women from seeking treatment at the hands of a white doctor.

The reporter concludes that the "flap underscores the difficulties and sensitivities of trying to reach out to minorities who are uncomfortable with, or distrustful of, the white-dominated medical system. Minority groups have a long history of being neglected by the mainstream medical system, and suspicions linger—particularly in the areas of genetic screening, one objective of the Sloan-Kettering study."[4]

Perhaps, as this book has suggested all along, racial memory is long and there are no easy ways—only better ways—to disseminate health care messages.

NOTES

1. AP Online, "Medicare No Longer a Sacred Cow," Prodigy Services Co., 26 June 1997, and "Medicare Changes May Fight Waste," Prodigy Services Co., 27 June 1997.

2. AP Online, "Shift to Managed Care is Inevitable," Prodigy Services Co., 2 July 1997

3. Lucette Lagnado, "When Racial Sensitivities Clash with Research." *The Wall Street Journal,* 25 June 1997, sec. B, p. 1.

4. Ibid

5. Ibid

Directing Health Messages toward African Americans

CHAPTER I

Introduction

Two people in different parts of the same city wake up in the morning not feeling well. Whether either seeks medical care depends on a variety of factors. Whether either has insurance or money to pay for a visit to a physician may make a difference. Difficulty in obtaining transportation to the doctor may matter. Whether either has knowledge about what his or her particular symptoms mean may be a factor. The decision may hinge on the ability to take time off from work or to arrange child care. Even their general attitudes toward the health care system, physicians, and their own health can influence their actions. Finally, whether one is an African American and the other a Caucasian can make a big difference in whether, how, and when they seek treatment; and race may also affect the quality of treatment they receive.

In short, a variety of factors influence health care, especially for African Americans. The literature clearly shows that poverty is extremely important. Poor people, in general, have more health problems and are more likely to die from preventable or easily treatable diseases. However, even when economics are comparable for the two groups, African Americans are generally in poorer health than any other racial group in America.

Although much research has been done on barriers to health care and on patient treatment and outcomes based on economic status and race, little has been done in regard to looking at the health care system from the patient's point of view. This study is concerned with two major subjects: attitudes toward the health care system and attitudes toward sources of health information from the individual's point of view. Furthermore, similarities and differences among minority and non-minority groups are studied to determine if some health messages can be more effectively transmitted to minority groups if they originate from certain sources, or if minority and non-minority individuals react similarly to health care messages.

A multi-dimensional approach to the communication of health messages is required to accomplish this. First, the author defines the scope of health care problems, particularly those affecting African Americans. Second, relevant communication and marketing theories are examined with emphasis placed on social marketing techniques. Third, research techniques, particularly Q methodology, are used to segment a mass audience along attitudinal, rather than demographic, lines. Fourth, strategies for the effective planning and dispersing of health messages are devised.

Q methodology and social marketing techniques are used to segment the mass audience and then evaluate attitudes and beliefs (along with some knowledge), particularly of minorities, in regard to health care information. The goals are to determine media exposure and attention to health care messages, the role of opinion leaders and societal factors, perceptions about health care availability and quality, and the impact of education and economic factors on behaviors for each of the various segments isolated.

Specifically, the research will focus on the differences between African Americans and Caucasians, especially in urban areas of Missouri and Louisiana, concerning how they obtain and act upon the health care information they receive. Among the questions to be addressed are: Do blacks and whites differ regarding media or societal influences? Is media exposure as important as economic factors regarding attitudes toward health care? Are opinion leaders of more importance to blacks than to whites?

The ultimate purpose of this research is to determine how to best plan health campaigns aimed at minorities in urban areas. More effective health care campaigns of this type are desirable for a number of reasons. First, research conducted in Missouri indicates that African Americans are more at risk than whites for several health concerns (such as cancer, infant mortality rates, high blood pressure, sickle cell anemia, and lupus). Additional national research shows that a higher proportion of African Americans delay treatment until their diseases become life-threatening or more costly to maintain. They also engage in lifestyles (i.e., higher consumption of cigarettes and alcohol and lower consumption rates of low-fat foods) that are more conducive to ill-health. Also, public health issues currently are high on the agendas of the political system, the public, and the media, which makes research into attitudes toward the health care system timely. Finally, it is the interest of every tax payer to decrease health costs by finding ways to increase prevention measures that could reduce the incidents of cancer, heart disease, stroke and other debilitating diseases in the American population.

To accomplish the research goals of this study, the author first turns to medical literature that defines the scope of the health care discrepancy between African Americans and the rest of the population and discusses many of the barriers that prevent minorities from seeking health care. The literature shows that morbidity and mortality rates differ between blacks and whites. Although most studies isolate poverty as the root cause of these discrepancies, other studies suggest availability of health care services, knowledge of how to use health care services, cultural attitudes, behaviors, and racism are also important factors. These studies are summarized in Chapter II.

Next, a review of relevant communication theories, focusing specifically on knowledge gaps, uses and gratifications, diffusion of information, and network analysis, is summarized in Chapter III. Also discussed are theories about media effects on mass audiences. Building on communication theory is a review of relevant information campaign literature, summarized in Chapter IV.

African American media habits also are important to this study. Although this is an area where research is in short supply, some pertinent studies are summarized in Chapter V.

Chapter VI describes the data collection methodology used in this study. First is a discussion of the focus groups used to isolate attitude statements which were used in the Q sort phase. Q methodology is explained in general, along with its specific application for this study. The rationale and description of methodology for a large-sample telephone survey conducted in St. Louis, Kansas City, and Baton Rouge are outlined in this chapter.

The five Q types that were obtained through factor analysis of the subjects who completed the Q sorts are described in Chapter VII. Chapter VIII summarizes the telephone survey results by clusters (based on Q types), and Chapter IX compares African American and Caucasian responses.

Chapter X draws conclusions and suggests possible strategies for designing health care campaigns aimed at minorities.

HYPOTHESES

The hypotheses which undergird this study are concerned with audience segmentation, sources of health care information, and perceived barriers to health care. They are as follows:

H1: Attitudes about health care are not unidimensional. The target audience can be segmented into definable groups of people who hold similar attitudes. Members of each group will have attitudes that are distinct from every other group.

H2: Not all African Americans think alike about health care. African American attitudes about health care will be represented by more than one clearly identifiable target audience segment.

H3: Media exposure and reliance patterns will not be uniform across all segments. Some audience segments are expected to be exposed more to print media (newspapers and magazines) than to broadcast media (radio and television), while the reverse will be true for other segments.

H4: Media sources will be more influential than interpersonal sources in the delivery of health care messages.

H5: Concerns about the health care system and recognition of barriers to obtaining health care will not be uniform across all segments.

CHAPTER II

African American Health Problems

Medical literature offers much proof that the health of African Americans in the United States is well below that of Americans of European descent and in many cases below that of Americans of Hispanic and Asian descent. Although the literature offers documentation of the problem, a wide variety of reasons are offered. Many researchers conclude that low socioeconomic conditions are at the root of the problem, but others have pointed out that when statistical controls are applied, African Americans still are more prone to disease than are their white counterparts in the same socioeconomic strata.

Most studies also rule out genetic reasons and point to a number of barriers, such as lack of access to health care professionals and facilities; the lack of trained African American health care practitioners—especially physicians; cultural insensitivity; and the lack of patient knowledge about illness prevention, especially nutrition. A few dare to suggest that discrimination remains at the heart of the matter.[1]

Schwartz et al. provide several statistics that show African Americans do not have access to adequate health care services:

Twenty percent of blacks do not have a regular source of health care and 22% do not have health insurance.[2] Among whites, the comparable numbers are 16% and 14% respectively. In addition, blacks are four times more likely than whites to rely on emergency rooms and hospital clinics for health services.[3] A similar trend is observed among low-income individuals, irrespective of race, who must postpone seeking primary care until their need for treatment becomes urgent and who then turn to hospital emergency rooms.[4]

7

This chapter will summarize some of the pertinent research concerning black health care both for Missouri—the focus of much of the research for this book—and for the nation.

AFRICAN AMERICAN HEALTH IN MISSOURI

In 1991, science writer Eric Adler compiled a four-part series on black health in Missouri for the Kansas City Star. His series begins:

> Pick an illness.
> Pick a disease
> Pick almost any medical horror, and odds are black people in the Kansas City area are afflicted at a rate of about 2-to-1 over white people. Liver disease. Cancers. Kidney disease. Diabetes. Infant death. Stroke.[5]

Adler writes that although death rates and incidence of disease for whites continue to drop, those for blacks began to climb again in the late 1980s. The reasons have little to do with genetic differences and much to do with problems ranging from poverty to blatant racism. Although life expectancy for whites has increased to 75 years, it has declined for blacks and is now 69 years. (For black males, it has dropped to less than 65.)

Adler points out that aside from human suffering, an unhealthy population means higher taxes and medical insurance premiums. He quotes Dr. Jasper Fullard Jr., a physician of internal medicine and president of Kansas City's Black Health Care Coalition: "If people aren't interested in this from the standpoint of humanity, they better start looking at the effect it's having financially."[6]

Adler writes that, reflecting national figures, Kansas City statistics reveal the following inequalities. Between 1980 and 1989, deaths among African Americans jumped 10 percent although they dropped 17 percent for white citizens. Cancer deaths were up 25 percent for blacks, but they were unchanged for whites. Deaths from heart disease—unchanged for blacks—dropped 28 percent for whites. Deaths resulting from diabetes, although increasing 16 percent for whites, increased 200 percent for blacks. During a 17- month period in 1990 and 1991, seven infants in the Kansas City area, all African American, were born with syphilis, compared with only four cases in the 1980s.[7]

Adler also writes that a review of patients with severe kidney disease between 1977 and 1985 found that blacks accounted for 33 percent of those with the disease but only got 21 percent of the kidney transplants, even though they were covered by Medicare. He says research confirms that black people are four to five times more likely than white people to have glaucoma, which is a leading cause of blindness. A national survey of patients discharged from hospitals with a diagnosis of anterior myocardial infarction, a type of heart attack, found the rate of diagnosis in black men was three-fourths that of white men. Nonetheless, black men were only one-third as likely to receive bypass surgery. A pneumonia study looked at all patients between 1970 and 1973 who were diagnosed with the illness at 17 selected hospitals. It found black patients were less likely to receive equal medical services, particularly intensive care.[8]

Adler reports that the U.S. Department of Health and Human Services estimates that of the 140,000 black people who die each year, about 60,000 are excess deaths—meaning that those blacks die of causes that would not have killed them had their health care been equal to that of whites. Of the 60,000 excess deaths, more than one-third are directly related to poverty, says the federal Centers for Disease Control in Atlanta. Nearly another third are a result of smoking, high blood pressure, high cholesterol level, obesity, alcohol consumption, diabetes, and lifestyle factors often related to income levels.[9]

Adler's series goes on to address the following issues associated with black health[10]:

1. **Racism and the stress of discrimination.** The effects of racism on darker-skinned blacks may be greater than the effects on those with lighter skin. A study of 186 black adults age 25 to 55 from Tuscaloosa, Ala., found the incidence of high blood pressure was 24 percent among darker-skinned persons compared with 7 percent of lighter-skinned subjects. Other experts blame racism for creating poor self-esteem and a physical depression that affects health.

2. **Poverty.** The National Research Council reported in 1989 that poverty may be "the most profound and pervasive" factor affecting the health disadvantages of blacks. Nearly one in three black residents in the Kansas City area lives beneath the poverty line and without money, people can't afford those things that promote a healthy life such as safe

housing, nutritious foods, leisure time for exercise, good transportation, medicines, safety devices to prevent injuries, quality education, or medical insurance.

3. **Biased care.** "Despite the progress of the past 25 years, racial prejudice has not been entirely eliminated in this country," the AMA's Council on Ethical and Judicial Affairs wrote in a 1990 issue of the *Journal of the American Medical Association.* "The health care system, like all elements of society has not fully eradicated this prejudice."

4. **AIDS.** Acquired immune deficiency syndrome continues to increase among African Americans. Although black Americans make up about 27% of the population in Kansas City, they represent 34% of all new AIDS cases. In the Kansas City area, heterosexual contact with individuals who trade sex for drugs, mostly crack, is more to blame (than sharing HIV-contaminated needles).

5. **Drugs.** The drug epidemic has hit hardest in areas where the black population is concentrated (60% are in metro areas and central cities). Drug use has had a major impact on child health and infant health and is strongly implicated in shooting deaths among young black men. Drug use also plays a role in liver disease and births of crack babies, many of whom are premature and wrought with developmental problems.

6. **Murder.** During the past decade, homicide was the leading killer of black male teen-agers in Kansas City. Recent state Health Department figures show murder isn't just the leading killer of black males between the ages of 15 and 24 but of all black males and females from ages 1 to 35. At least 85% of homicides in the Kansas City area are blacks killing blacks.

7. **Access to care.** About 22% of all black people have no medical coverage—public or private. About 12% of white people have no coverage. Without money or any type of medical insurance, many people delay getting care until they are very ill. In a national AMA survey, one of every 11 black people reported not seeing a doctor in 1986 because they could not pay. That compared with one in 20 whites.

8. **Infants and children.** Black babies are twice as likely to be born underweight and to die before their first birthday. The overall death rate for black children is 30% to 50% higher than for whites. The homicide rate among young black children is almost four times that of white children. It is the second leading cause of death, behind accidents.

Malnutrition, anemia, lead poisoning, lack of immunization, child abuse and neglect are more likely among black children.

9. **Young adults.** The death rate for young black people is about 30% higher than for white people. Black mothers die from complications during pregnancy or childbirth at a rate three times that of whites. Homicide is the leading killer of black youths and young adults aged 15 to 24, with a rate seven times that of whites. The death rate from AIDS is 15 times higher for black women aged 25 to 34 than for white females. For black men, it's three times greater than the death rate for white men.

10. **Older Adults.** The death rate for black adults aged 45 to 64 is about 75% higher than for white adults. For black females aged 65 to 74, the death rate from heart disease is 60% higher. The death rate from stroke is 111% higher. About 80% of black people over age 55 have hypertension, compared with about 65% of white people. For black men aged 55 to 64, the overall cancer death rate is 47% higher than for white men.

In another major study of racial differences in cancer mortality in Missouri, Brownson, Davis and Chang report that in 1990 the discrepancy between black and white cancer mortality rates in the state remains a cause of concern for the public health community. Cancer is the second leading cause of death in Missouri, accounting for 10,913 deaths in 1988.[11]

The researchers say that "although cancer is a serious public health concern for all segments of the population, it impacts certain racial groups more severely"[12] and that African Americans have the highest overall cancer mortality rate among the major racial and ethnic groups in the United States.[13] (National data suggest that cancer mortality rates are 27% higher among blacks than whites.)[14]

The researchers also say:

The age-adjusted mortality rate per 100,000 for all cancer sites combined was 210 among white males, and 313 among black males. The corresponding rates in white and black females were 132 and 178, respectively. These rates represent a white-black difference in total cancer mortality of 49% for males and 35% for females. . . . The average annual lung cancer rate was 32% higher among black men than white men and

23% higher among black women than white women. Racial differences by age group among males were greatest in the younger age groups, whereas white-black differences in female lung cancer rates were relatively constant over all age groups.

Age-specific rates of colorectal cancer were higher for black men than any other race or sex subgroup in each age group. Colorectal cancer rates were 43% higher for black women than white women and 34% higher for black men than white men.

The largest racial difference in cancer rates was noted for prostate cancer. The overall, age-adjusted prostate cancer rate for blacks was 41.5 per 100,000, compared with 19.8 per 100,000 for white. This is a difference of 110%.[15]

The study concludes that Missouri cancer mortality rates among blacks are higher than those among whites for all cancer sites combined and for each of the four major cancer types (i.e., lung, colorectal, prostate, and breast) studied. Differences between white and black total cancer mortality in Missouri are larger than national estimates for both males (49% in Missouri vs. 38% in the U.S.[16]) and females (35% in Missouri vs. 14% in the U.S.[17]).

They point to higher rates of smoking among African Americans compared to whites as a major and preventable contributing factor. Other cancer risk factors of concern in black populations include alcohol consumption (heavy drinking is more common among African Americans), nutrition, and occupational exposures.[18] Dietary factors account for an estimated 35% of all cancer deaths;[19] however, few detailed data have been collected on racial differences in dietary patterns. Furthermore, limited information is available on occupational exposures, though blacks are more likely to be employed in occupations that place them at higher risk for cancer.[20]

The researchers also find that the tendency toward the later disease stage at the time of diagnosis among blacks for the cancers studied is a "clear contributor to the higher cancer mortality rates in blacks. . . . (In the study) 15% fewer blacks than whites were diagnosed at the localized stage, and 14% more blacks than whites had distant disease."[21]

Two other researchers, Mayer and McWhorter, point out that decreased survival in black patients relative to white patients with bladder cancer has been documented in several reports. Factors contributing to this survival difference include: age, diagnosis at more advanced stages, and more aggressive tumor histology. Blacks continue to have poorer five-year relative survival rates.[22]

Brownson et al. found that lower socioeconomic status was an important predictor of the high cancer mortality among blacks.[23] The percentage of black Americans below the poverty level (33.8%) is three times that for white Americans (11.5%). The researchers conclude:

> Lower socioeconomic status affects other factors that influence cancer survival, such as knowledge of primary prevention, knowledge and availability of early detection practices, and access to state-of-the-art treatment. For example, survey data suggest that blacks tend to accept common cancer myths more readily (e.g., bruising causes cancer), that they may delay as much as three to 12 months before seeking treatment, and that they have a more pessimistic attitude toward cancer survival.[24]

AFRICAN AMERICAN HEALTH NATIONWIDE

A number of other studies around the country have documented the extensive health care problems that African Americans face. These studies have ranged from barriers and problems of access to disease-specific diagnoses and treatment problems. The following is a summary of the studies relevant to this research.

BARRIERS TO HEALTH CARE

In an editorial in the New York State Journal of Medicine (1991), Dr. Victor W. Sidel wrote:

> It is well known that the most important determinants of health or illness are the economic, social, and physical environments in which people live rather than the quality of their medical care or even the quality of their conventionally defined health care.[25]

Sidel lists several ways in which people living in inner cities are "victimized." These include inadequate housing, hunger and malnutrition, pressure from advertising and peers to use harmful substances (tobacco, alcohol and illegal drugs), hazards in the workplace and environment (lead levels, pollutants) and racism which denies equal opportunity and sets up risks. But, he points to poverty as the "overarching victimization":

> One-fourth of all children under the age of five in the United States live below the officially designated "poverty line" and one half of all African American children under the age of five live below that level. Furthermore, the poverty line is purposely set low to hide the magnitude of the problem and millions of children and adults who are forced to live at levels 50% or 100% above the line may also be in terrible need.[26]

The health consequences of these living conditions also are well known, he said. These consequences include more low birthweight babies; higher neonatal, post-neonatal, and childhood mortality rates; infectious diseases preventable by immunization; learning and behavioral disorders resulting from poor nutrition, homelessness, and blood lead levels; asthma and other breathing disorders associated with environmental pollution; injury and death from violence; and nephrologic problems.[27]

Petchers and Milligan stress that providing access to a minimum level of health care for traditionally disadvantaged groups continues to be an important public-policy concern. They cite such barriers as transportation problems, fragmentation and depersonalization, long waiting times and inconvenient hours of service at health care facilities, a confusing clinic or hospital atmosphere, and not seeing the same physician twice. They also cite studies that pinpoint insensitivity of doctors and nurses, a lack of effective communications, patient fears of doctors and hospitals, fear of diagnosis or prognosis and lack of faith in the medical profession as additional barriers.[28] However, Gylys and Gylys find that lower income blacks do not have negative attitudes toward medical institutions or the medical profession. They, in fact, tend to have considerable trust in medical care and believe they will receive quality care.[29]

Petchers and Milligan conclude that affordability is a formidable barrier to medical care for the sample of poor, minority elderly who had difficulty meeting medical expenses despite high enrollment rates in Medicare and Medicaid.[30]

In an editorial in *Diabetes Care*, Anderson et al. report on barriers to diabetes care identified by a University of Michigan Diabetes Research and Training Center Task Force on Diabetes and the Black Population in 1990.

The force was formed to "identify potential barriers to the translation of scientific knowledge into improved health care and health for blacks with diabetes."[31] The potential barriers prove to be: racism, lack of knowledge, incorrect beliefs, lack of access to health care, differing cultural values and priorities, and poverty—all of which are interrelated.

The authors say that the limited progress made in reducing institutional racism has in some ways made life more difficult for individual blacks because they must confront the erroneous belief held by many white Americans that the failure of many blacks to succeed now is because of their own inferiority rather than the result of racism.[32]

Anderson et al. point out that although most daily diabetes care is in the hands of the patient, the gap between essential information and patients' actual knowledge may be greater for blacks with diabetes than for whites in part due to the lack of culturally sensitive patient education programs and materials for blacks.[33]

Traditionally, education programs have been developed by white professionals for white patients, Hopper says. The same diabetes education program presented by the same health professional may be perceived quite differently by black and nonwhite people.[34]

Anderson et al. add:

Many of the programs and materials created specifically for African Americans have been developed by layering ethnic applications onto pre-existing programs. The failure of many white health care professionals to understand the culture of their black patients may also contribute to this discrepancy.

Health behavior is strongly influenced by cultural patterns. When health professionals and patients are from different ethnic and cultural backgrounds, they may have different beliefs and expectations about health behaviors. Conflict and educational and communication failures may result from these differences.[35]

The authors elaborate on this by pointing out that many white health care professionals do not understand or appreciate differences in the use of the English language by many blacks (different pronunciations, different meanings). Body language between blacks and whites also can be a barrier.

Black people may move in close while talking and look away while listening.[36]

The authors said that the black culture has an active folk medicine system comprised of European folklore, classic medicine, and current medicine. Hopper says that health professionals might not recognize that African Americans may try folk remedies first or in combination with orthodox treatment because they do not fit in with the traditional medical model.[37]

Anderson et al. also emphasize that within the African American community there is a strong "sense of the present" that may make looking toward the future, planning, and preventive health measure inconsistent with their views.[38] Therefore, some black patients may be difficult to convince to care for their diabetes today to prevent future complications.

The editorial suggests that health beliefs also are affected by how people perceive their ability to control their lives or fates. Members of minority groups, particularly older people, may exhibit a fatalistic or helpless attitude. If people believe there is little that they can do to influence their health they may not seek treatment or follow prescribed treatment plans.[39]

Anderson et al. warn that exploring the values and attitudes of the poor and of blacks is controversial because it is reminiscent of previous debates concerning the "culture of poverty." They say:

> Implicit in the culture of poverty argument is the notion that the problems of low-income minorities are created by minorities themselves. It is argued that these deficiencies are the results of deep-seated cultural values and could not be easily modified. It is unclear whether the impact of poverty on diabetes care is the same for people of all races or whether there are race-specific barriers that affect black people regardless of their socioeconomic standing. Although it is known that many blacks are poor, it is a mistake to equate blackness with poverty.[40]

The central question, they said, is the relationship among knowledge, attitudes, beliefs, and socioeconomic status and use of services within the black population.[41]

ACCESS

Blendon et al. conducted a national survey concerning the use of health services. Their findings include a "significant deficit" in access to health care among African Americans compared with white Americans. This gap is experienced by all income levels of black Americans. The study also finds significant under-use by blacks of needed medical care. Moreover, blacks compared with whites, are less likely to be satisfied with the qualitative ways their physicians treat them when they are ill, more dissatisfied with the care they receive when hospitalized and more likely to believe that the duration of their hospitalizations is too short.[42]

The Department of Health and Human Services' Secretary's Task Force on Black and Minority Health report black Americans continue to have a 1½ times higher death rate than whites of the same age, and the infant mortality rate for blacks is twice that of whites.[43]

Given the disparity between white and black health, it is of considerable concern that the 1986 national survey of 10,130 persons living in the continental United States found a significant deficit remains in access to health care among blacks, compared with white Americans. Although Blendon et al. point out that social and cultural differences among population groups also are related to health care behavior, the volume of care received by low-income populations is highly sensitive both to the presence of financial barriers to health care and to the availability of medical resources in the community.[44]

The survey finds blacks worse off than whites in terms of access to physician care with blacks having a significantly higher rate than whites of not seeing a physician within a one-year period (37.2% compared with 31.7%). The average annual number of physician visits among blacks compared with whites also is lower (3.4 per year compared with 4.4). Also the study finds lower access to health care of blacks compared with whites even when health status is taken into account. The researchers say a key issue is whether differences are explainable by the well-documented income differential between blacks and whites in the United States or the fact that blacks on the average are younger than the white population. A multiple regression analyses finds that even after taking into account persons' income, health status, age, sex, and whether they had one or more chronic or serious illnesses, blacks have a statistically significantly lower mean number of annual ambulatory visits and are less likely to have seen a physician in a year.[45]

The 1986 survey clearly establishes that there is significant underuse of medical care by African Americans. One in 11 African Americans who report they have one of ten chronic or serious illnesses about which they were specifically questioned did not have an ambulatory visit in the year preceding the survey, compared with one in six white persons surveyed. Among persons reporting they have hypertension, 30% of blacks have not had an annual blood pressure check compared with 19% of whites. The differences between whites and blacks in use of health services also extend to dental care with about 50% of blacks, compared with 36% of whites, receiving no dental care in the year prior to the survey.[46]

The researchers conclude that in part, the black-white differences reflect the indirect consequences of economic level of living, but ethnic-related differences in health care arrangements and life-style also are important.

They find that not only are African Americans less likely to have any insurance coverage, they are considerably less likely to be covered by a private insurance carrier (85.1% compared with 72.5%). Blacks are significantly more likely to reside in Southern and Southwestern states with the least generous Medicaid programs.[47]

Almost half of the African Americans surveyed had used hospital clinics, emergency departments, community health centers, or other organized settings for their last visit (if they had a visit in the past year) compared with only slightly more than one-fourth of whites. African Americans also are significantly more likely than whites to prefer to go to a different provider for their health care than they saw at their last visit.

The researchers also suggest that the undersupply of black physicians and of physicians in general in minority communities also may result in reduced opportunities for medical care.[48]

Finally, the researchers acknowledge that some cultural differences between blacks and whites could explain some of the differences they found:

> The survey did not include measures that directly reflect black-white cultural differences that might explain the access findings reported. However, the differences in health care arrangements just discussed are persistent features of the sociocultural milieux of the two racial groups. Consequently, it is a reasonable conjecture that underlying some of our

findings are unmeasured sociocultural differences between blacks and whites that are associated with the findings on access to care.[49]

Findings regarding patient satisfaction is also worth mentioning. African Americans are more likely than whites to report that on their last visit, their physician did not inquire sufficiently about pain, did not tell them how long it would take for prescribed medicine to work, did not explain the seriousness of the illness or injury, and did not discuss test or examination findings. Moreover, African Americans are less satisfied with the care received both while hospitalized and during ambulatory visits. Fewer than three-fifths of blacks are completely satisfied with care provided during their last hospitalization, compared with more than three-fourths of whites. Blacks also are more likely than whites to wait for more than half an hour before seeing a physician at their last ambulatory visit.[50]

WOMEN AND HEALTH INSURANCE

Braveman et al. focus on the problem of lack of health insurance for women, a problem that is particularly severe for women of ethnic minorities who are over-represented among poor women.

From 9% to 18% of the entire population has insufficient health insurance.[51] The figure of about 37 million persons, or 15% of the population, is widely accepted as a current estimate of those who are uninsured for all or part of a given year.[52] Further, women generally are more likely than men to be poor and to live longer.

The authors said that incomplete insurance coverage for minority women is of particular concern because minorities, especially black women, endure a disproportionate burden of illness and thus have greater needs for health care.[53] They write:

> Blacks in the United States have twice the rate of infant morality compared with whites.[54] Overall, age-adjusted mortality rates are higher for minority women than for their white counterparts.[55] While the incidence of breast cancer appears to be higher among white women, breast cancer survival raters are higher for white than for black women, who tend to be diagnosed at more advanced stages of disease.[56] Death rates from heart disease are twice as high for black as for white women. The black:white ratio for stroke morality in women is 2.5:1.[57] When compared with white women, black women also have higher mortality rates from cirrhosis and

diabetes mellitus and are at higher risk for tuberculosis, hypertension, and anemia.[58]

Braveman et al. say minority women are far more likely to be poor than their non-Latino white counterparts with one-third of blacks and more than a quarter of Latinos living in poverty. Compounding the problem is the fact that many insured women, including pregnant women with private or public coverage and elderly women, are underinsured. The authors conclude that relationships between women's poverty, health insurance coverage, and health status imply that those with the greatest health care needs are least likely to have financial access to care.

NONEMERGENCY VISITS TO EMERGENCY ROOMS

White-Means and Thornton have studied reasons why the emergency room, initially envisioned as a source of treatment for trauma and acute health conditions, has expanded its role to become a substitute for the physician, outpatient facility, and clinic.[59] They write:

> For an increasing number of patients, the emergency room now provides the only door of access to the mainstream health care system and has supplanted the traditional role of the physician's office. Thus, these patients consider the emergency room as their usual source of care, and it has become the so-called "community physician."[60]

In spite of difficulties such as long waiting times and discontinuity of care, the authors say several features of the emergency room make it an attractive source of primary health care for certain populations: use is not contingent on affiliation with a particular doctor; no appointment is needed to receive care; it provides immediate access to sophisticated medical technology, if needed; it has "office hours" that continue beyond the normal closing hours of other health care providers; and health-insurance policies generally provide unlimited access to its services.

The researchers say that although the extent of emergency room use is well-documented, sociodemographic determinants of its use remain unclear, particularly for non-emergency conditions. They report:

Descriptive data suggest that race, socioeconomic status, and the type of insurance coverage are each distinguishing features of emergency room users. These data show that blacks use the emergency room more frequently than whites and that emergency room users are more often of low socioeconomic status. Finally, [studies] have shown that use of the emergency room declines if the insurance policy requires patients to make out-of-pocket payments that represent a high percentage of the cost of emergency room care.

The predisposing conditions affecting emergency room visits by blacks and whites include household status, marital status, sex, age, and education.[61]

The researchers find that while educational status (college graduation) is a significant deterrent to emergency room visits by whites, it is an insignificant factor in visit decisions by blacks.

The researchers speculate that in black communities, the emergency room may be perceived as the only health care provider. If that is the case, economic factors (e.g., the availability of health insurance that reduces the relative prices of medical services) may not affect decision-making.[62]

The researchers also find that while single and widowed whites are significantly less likely than are those who are married to use medical services, marital status is an insignificant determinant of medical use by blacks. Widowhood, as compared to those who are married, is an insignificant determinant of emergency room use by whites and lowers the probability of emergency room use by blacks. They suggest that the role of family structure in influencing medical use decisions and facility choice is different across racial groups.[63]

The researchers say that economic factors are generally insignificant in explaining the emergency room use by blacks while they are highly significant for whites, but it is unclear whether these factors are related to cultural preference of blacks or characteristics of the communities in which black consumers receive medical services.[64] They concluded that there is need to distinguish cultural/ethnic factors from effects of racial discrimination and to determine if blacks' use patterns are influenced by cultural phenomena and/or by a realistic assessment of the assistance available to them.

LOW BIRTH WEIGHT

Infant mortality in the United States continues to be a worrisome public-health problem both because the rates are too high relative to other developed nations and because some minority groups, most especially African Americans, have much higher rates than whites.[65] According to Hale and Druschel, "Just as low birth weight is the most significant risk factor for neonatal mortality, poverty seems to be the major determinant of postneonatal death. Poverty may be defined in terms of familial characteristics or those of the community."[66]

The authors' study in Alabama found that white infants from rural areas have the highest neonatal mortality rates while black infants from rural areas have the highest postneonatal mortality rates and the highest rate of deaths due to infection, a potentially preventable cause of death. These infants also have greater numbers of deaths attributed to unknown causes.[67]

Scupholme et al. have studied the barriers that prevent women, from a multiethnic and primarily indigent urban population, from obtaining prenatal care. The results indicate that the main barriers were systematic (35.5%), patient-related (35.5%), and financial (29%). Ethnic group, marital status, and education influence access to prenatal care, whereas age does not appear to do so. It also is apparent that cultural behavior influenced babies' birth weight, whether or not prenatal care was obtained.[68]

Studies indicate that mothers who come from low socioeconomic backgrounds are most likely to receive inadequate prenatal care and to produce low birth weight babies.[69] Poor financial resources, patient attitudes, and structural barriers in the prenatal care system are the main obstacles to receive adequate prenatal care. African American women showed not only the highest percentage of low birth weight babies within ethnic groups, but also 50% of the low birth weight babies came from 32% of the population.[70] National statistics have shown that black women have a low birth weight rate that is twice that of the white population.[71]

Scupholme et al. find that African American women have much higher rates of low birth weight babies regardless of prenatal care, whereas women from Haiti and the Caribbean islands have rates that are similar to the white population. They conclude that this difference within the black population needs further research to assess any cultural influencing factors other than ethnicity, low socioeconomic status, or prenatal care.[72]

The researchers say most women in the study sample stated that they believe prenatal care is important for the health of mother and baby. However, neither proximity to the clinic nor knowledge of the clinic location is indicative that a mother will access the prenatal care system. Therefore, the researchers conclude that there remains a need for more education about the benefits of prenatal care and for identifying which aspects of prenatal care are important to each cultural group with more emphasis placed on incorporating cultural belief systems into prenatal care "because belief in the importance of care is not sufficient to lead to action."[73]

Some women with previous experiences in clinics, cited long waits, staff attitudes, and inconvenient hours as reasons for not obtaining prenatal care.[74]

DIABETES

Only 5.8 million of the estimated 11 million cases of diabetes have been diagnosed by a physician.[75] Direct medical costs of diabetes are about $7.4 billion annually, and indirect costs, such as lost productivity, total another $6.3 billion. Estimates by the American Diabetes Association indicate that diabetes is twice as common among African Americans aged 45 to 65 as among whites in the same age-group and three times more common after age 65.[76]

Anderson et al. summarizes statistics that show the prevalence of diabetes is substantially higher among blacks than whites:

> Black men have a rate that is 1.4 times higher than white men, and black women have a rate ~2 times higher than white women. During the 1980s, age-standardized mortality for white men and women declined 1.6 and 4.5%, respectively, although among black men and women, mortality increased 11 and 5.5%, respectively. In 1987, the age-adjusted rate of 183 hospitalizations related to diabetes/10,000 black women was 36% higher than for black men (135/10,000), 95% higher than for white women (94/10,000), and 108% higher than for white men (88/10,000). In 1987, the age-adjusted rate of hospital discharges for diabetic ketoacidosis among black men with diabetes was 24.7/1000. This was nearly threefold higher than the corresponding rate of 8.7/1000 white men with diabetes. Similar discrepancies exist between black and white women with diabetes.[77]

The authors also say that when end-stage renal disease incidence is calculated with diabetic population denominators, the rates for black men and women are more than twice those for white men and women.[78] They also find that hospital discharge rates for lower- extremity amputation are consistently higher for blacks with diabetes than for whites with diabetes.[79] They conclude that African Americans are at increased risk for both diabetes and its complications—many of which are preventable through behavioral changes and preventative health care services.[80]

Physicians also may bear some responsibility for poor patient outcomes. One study the authors cite indicates that physicians with predominantly black or Hispanic patient populations are significantly less likely to recommend preventive practices and screening tests compared with physicians with predominantly white patient populations.[81]

Davidson provides additional reasons for the higher incident rate in the African American population. Minority groups have excess morbidity and mortality related to gestational diabetes possibly because minority women may not see a physician until late in their pregnancies. There could be a genetic susceptibility for type II diabetes. Obesity is a risk factor for type II diabetes, and African Americans tend to have a higher rate of obesity than does the general population. Related to obesity is a sedentary lifestyle. Although exercise improves both glucose tolerance and increases insulin secretion, it is not emphasized as much in some ethnic groups as it is in others, particularly for persons who are middle-aged or older.[82]

Davidson also emphasizes that all low-income groups share a lack of access to continuing, high-quality, affordable medical care:

> Decades of poor health care result in a heavy burden of chronic disorders, including obesity, hypertension, diabetes, and associated complications. Over the last 20 years, diabetes-related mortality and morbidity have increased, as have costs for late-stage diabetes care. When health care does come to low-income areas (e.g., through health fairs or other short-term programs), patients are usually lost to follow-up care even if their diabetes is diagnosed.[83]

NEUROLOGICAL CARE

In a 1991 article, Kenton focuses on the lack of access to neurological care for minorities. He points out that it is well-documented that access to health care is dependent on one's socioeconomic level and that minorities comprise the majority of the lower socioeconomic scale.[84] Minorities comprise a large component of the estimated 34 to 37 million Americans under age 65 who have no health care insurance.[85] Life expectancy among many minority groups has declined in recent years, while mortality rates among the poor and disadvantaged are higher for most causes of death as are prevalence rates of major disabilities including heart disease, cancer, and stroke.[86]

Numerous studies reveal that approximately 28% of adult blacks suffer from hypertension compared with about 17% of adult whites and that blacks develop hypertension at a younger age than do whites. Advanced hypertension is five times more common in blacks. Stroke mortality in blacks is 65% higher than that in whites. Black persons with hypertension probably are more susceptible than are hypertensive whites to the neurologic complications of the disease. Although whites and blacks respond similarly to antihypertensive therapy, minority populations do not receive the therapy to the same degree as the white population because of access-limiting costs of drugs, continuity of care, early intervention, and education of drug effects.[87]

Kenton points out that early treatment can reduce the complications of heart disease, cancer, and stroke damage to the central nervous system; but to disadvantaged minorities, neurologic symptoms and signs as well as the discipline itself are enigmas. He said minority patients may refuse a lumbar puncture for fear of paralysis or fear of spreading the malady, or equate multiple sclerosis with muscular dystrophy or refuse scans or imaging of the brain for fear of brain injury. Others fail to initiate or maintain medication due to cost.[88]

In addition, Kenton said, many minority senior citizens supported by Medicare and adequate supplementary insurance could afford a private doctor; but they often are admitted from emergency rooms to the teaching services as unassigned patients to be followed thereafter by residents in the outpatient clinics. This practice limits their access to more experienced physicians. Kenton concludes that minorities, regardless of economics, because of limited contact with physicians of their own background and because of low rates of preventive physical examinations continue to lag behind the nation's norms in access.[89]

In the *American Journal of Medicine*, Haywood reports that data from multiple sources confirm the greater risk of morbidity and mortality from cardiovascular disease that is seen in some minority segments of the population of the United States, when those segments are compared with the population as a whole. In most studies, African Americans have higher overall mortality rates from cardiovascular disease than Hispanics and substantially higher rates than whites and Asians. In some of these studies, African Americans also have higher rates of both hypertension-related stroke and coronary artery disease. Issues related to access to care may affect the disproportionate morbidity and mortality rates found in African American and Hispanic patients, as well as among some lower-class segments of the non-Hispanic white population. Haywood said access to care may depend upon a number of factors, such as cultural isolation, public awareness, individual and group attitudes, perception of resource availability, actual resources, socioeconomic status, educational level, and peer behavior.[90] Thus, access to care "can be defined in terms of the availability and quality of health facilities—and, after that, the attitudinal and socioeconomic factors that tend to limit (or encourage) the use of such facilities."[91]

CANCER

Cancer is the second leading cause of death among African Americans, responsible for 53,968 deaths in 1988. Only heart disease exceeds cancer as a cause of mortality.[92]

Boring et al. report that cancer incidence rates are nearly twice as high or higher for African Americans compared with whites for cancers of the esophagus, uterus, cervix, liver, and stomach and for multiple myeloma.[93] They concluded that some of these increased rates are due to socioeconomic differences such as dietary patterns, alcohol use, and sexual and reproductive behaviors.

A 1990 study from the National Cancer Institute presented black and white cancer rates by socioeconomic status. The authors report:

> . . . for all cancer sites combined, cancer incidence was higher in low-education and low-income groups regardless of race. When rates were statistically adjusted for income or education, cancer rates for whites were

higher than for blacks. Specific sites associated with low income in both races were lung and uterine cervix. Breast cancer in white women was related to higher levels of income and education. Prostate, stomach, and cervical cancer rates were higher among blacks even after adjustment for income or education. This analysis demonstrates that many cancers diagnosed more frequently among blacks do not reflect racial predisposition but are a consequence of cultural factors.[94]

Mayer and McWhorter's study, using as an indicator the proportion untreated, indicates that there are differences in treatment status between black and white bladder cancer patients. Black patients were more than twice as likely as white patients to go untreated. This difference was only partially explained by racial differences in age at diagnosis, stage at diagnosis, sex, or tumor histology.[95]

HEART DISEASE

Coronary heart disease (CHD) mortality rates for African Americans exceed those of whites at ages 25-64 and are similar to the rates of whites for all ages combined.[96] In contrast, population rates of CHD occurrence based on cases from hospital discharge surveys are lower for African Americans than for whites.[97] This inconsistency may be due to bias in detection and measurement, or it also might reflect an excess of CHD deaths among blacks before the hospital is reached. A study of CHD in Newark found that blacks are more likely to be dead on arrival at the hospital,[98] while a study in urban and rural areas of South Carolina reported that blacks have higher rates of out-of- hospital mortality from acute myocardial infarction.[99]

Strogatz reports that among those who do not die immediately, blacks and whites may differ by how quickly medical care follows the onset of symptoms. Blacks, compared to whites, are far less likely to be seen by a cardiologist, to have coronary angiography performed, and to undergo coronary artery bypass surgery, and these differences persist even among hospitalized patients, controlling for the clinical severity of disease.[100]

Strogatz also asserts that less is known about black-white differences in patients' knowledge of symptoms and decisions to seek care. Studies have found that blacks have low levels of knowledge about CHD, its signs and symptoms, are less informed about the symptoms of myocardial infarction and are more likely to delay in seeking treatment for myocardial infarction.[101]

The authors said these findings indicate that gaps in knowledge and delays in receiving care may contribute to black-white differences in pre-hospital mortality from CHD.

Strogatz indicates that other possible explanations for the black-white difference in medical care utilization include differences in perceptions about the seriousness of the symptom and the potential efficacy of medical care:

> Compared to whites, blacks may be less likely to perceive chest pain as serious enough to warrant immediate medical attention. Berkanovic and Telesky[102] suggest that the pronounced association between severity of symptoms and utilization for blacks may be a vestige of past circumstances in which only the most disabling conditions could serve as justification for interruption of one's duties in order to seek care. This habit may persist today even for individuals who have more resources or autonomy over their personal lives. Studies of whites with chest pain suggest that both the severity of the symptom and an individual's flexibility to respond at the time of symptom onset will contribute to delay in receiving care.[103]

Blacks and whites also may view the likely efficacy of visiting the doctor differently. Strogatz found that hypertensive black adults have less confidence in the net benefit of anti-hypertensive medication, and this attitude was associated with a greater likelihood of being untreated for diagnosed hypertension.[104]

DELAYED ACCESS TO HEALTH CARE

In 1991 Weissman et al. reported the results of their study undertaken to determine characteristics of patients reporting delays in care before hospitalization and the reasons for those delays. They found that delays in care were reported by 16% of all patients. The odds of reporting delays in care among patients who were black, poor, uninsured, or without a regular physician were 40% to 80% greater than those for other patients. Patients reporting delays most often thought their medical problem was not serious (64%), but cost was an important factor for patients in lower socioeconomic positions. The odds of delaying care because of cost for patients who were both poor and uninsured were 12 times greater than the odds for other patients. In addition, patients who reported delays had 9% longer hospital stays compared with others (after controlling for diagnosis-related groups and severity).[105]

Patients may experience delays in obtaining care for illnesses that eventually lead to hospitalization for various reasons, the researchers found:

> (Patients) may fail to recognize the symptoms of significant medical problems that require attention or may encounter financial and organizational barriers that particularly affect disadvantaged populations. Such delays may result in the patient being more severely ill at admission and with a worse prognosis, and possibly a longer hospital stay and higher costs than if he or she had received care earlier. Facilitating the timely and appropriate use of health services may therefore improve health status and perhaps decrease costs.[106]

They say that despite general agreement about the importance of seeking and receiving prompt medical attention for major illnesses, relatively little is known about the socio-economic and clinical characteristics of patients who experience delays, particularly for conditions that are serious enough to require hospitalization:

> Most studies of patients' reasons for delays in care have limited their field of inquiry to conceptual beliefs and coping styles, such as how well patients understood the nature of their disease or the expected course of their treatment. Surprisingly, financial barriers have received much less attention. To our knowledge, only one analysis has directly considered the cost of care as a factor in patients' delaying care, and no studies have shown the effect of delays in care on the ultimate cost of medical treatment.[107]

This study, as well as a number of other studies cited, show that patients who are black, poor, uninsured, or without a regular source of care may face impediments to access, as evidenced by lower use of health services. The authors suggest that access problems may be broader than previous studies have reported because even patients who eventually received care in hospitals may experience delays before treatment.[108]

TREATMENT DIFFERENCES BETWEEN
AFRICAN AMERICANS AND CAUCASIANS

Several studies have examined the difference in care and medical procedure between blacks and whites. Generally, the studies have found that African Americans are given fewer procedures and are dismissed from hospitals in less stable conditions than white patients.

The Council on Ethical and Judicial Affairs of the American Medical Association reported in 1989 that persistent, and sometimes substantial, differences continue to exist in the quality of health among Americans. Differences in both need and access underlie the disparities in the quality of health among Americans. Blacks are more likely to require health care but are less likely to receive health care services; and recent studies have suggested that even when blacks gain access to the health care system, they are less likely than whites to receive certain surgical or other therapies.

The Council emphasized the need for:

> (1) greater access to necessary health care for black Americans, (2) greater awareness among physicians of existing and potential disparities in treatment, and (3) the continued development of practice parameters, including criteria that would preclude or diminish racial disparities in health care decisions.

Recent studies suggest that the use of specific medical treatments differ between black and white patients. These studies have examined treatments in several areas, including cardiology and cardiac surgery, kidney transplantation, general internal medicine, and obstetrics.

A national survey found that black men have a rate of anterior myocardial infarction that was three fourths of the rate for white men. However, the black men are only half as likely to undergo angiography (a diagnostic procedure) and one third as likely to undergo bypass surgery as the white men even though mortality rates suggested that the severity of illness is comparable between blacks and whites at the time of admission.[109]

Another study of all patients discharged from Massachusetts hospitals in 1985 with a preliminary diagnosis of circulatory system disease or chest pain found that while blacks and whites have similar rates of hospitalization, whites are one-third more likely to undergo coronary angiography and more than twice as likely to be treated with bypass surgery or angioplasty. The racial disparities persist even after differences in income and the severity of disease are taken into account.[110]

The Council also reports that race correlates with the likelihood that a patient with kidney disease will receive long-term hemodialysis or a kidney transplant. Racial disparities in access to long-term hemodialysis are on the order of 5% to 15%.

The Council says evidence of racial disparities in treatment decisions also appears in general internal medicine. A study of treatment for patients hospitalized because of pneumonia found that the patient's race correlates with the intensity of care provided. The study shows that, after controlling for differences in clinical characteristics and income, blacks are less likely to receive medical services, particularly intensive care.[111]

The Council points out that racial disparities in treatment decisions have been documented previously, such as in a study that found blacks are more likely to be classified as ward patients and whites to be classified as private patients, even when there is a comparable ability to pay for care. Also, ward patients are less frequently admitted to the hospital even when clinical characteristics are similar.[112]

The Council says:

> It is difficult to draw firm conclusions from these studies regarding the role of race in decisions to treat patients. With regard to bypass surgery, for example, while the studies tried to control for incidence and severity of disease, they generally did not control for other relevant variables that may account for the differences between blacks and whites. . . .[113]

It suggests some of the disparity in kidney transplantation rates may be explained by medical or biologic differences. For example, most of the kidneys donated for transplantation come from whites, and intraracial antigen matching is often more favorable than interracial matching. However, the Council concludes it is unlikely that medical differences account for all of the disparities because income differences have a major effect. Race and income are highly correlated and patients with higher incomes are better able to bear the direct and indirect costs of expensive medical procedures.

The Council concludes:

> Some medical experts have also suggested that physicians are more likely to treat aggressively patients who are wealthier, more productively

employed, and more assertive. Such patients might be viewed as more likely to respond successfully to therapy. It has also been suggested that they might be viewed as more valuable to society.[114]

The Council emphasizes three approaches that it believes should be given high priority:

1. Greater access: The studies discussed in this report underscore the need for ensuring that black Americans without adequate health care insurance are given the means for access to necessary health care.
2. Greater awareness: Because racial disparities may be occurring despite the lack of any intent or purposeful efforts to treat patients differently on the basis of race, physicians should examine their own practices to ensure that inappropriate considerations do not affect their clinical judgment. . . .
3. Practice parameters: The racial disparities in treatment decisions indicate that inappropriate considerations may enter the decision-making process.[115]

Peterson et al. examines whether blacks admitted to Veterans Affairs Medical Centers with an acute myocardial infarction are less likely than whites to undergo cardiac catheterization and revascularization procedures. The Veterans Hospital Administration provides medical care to all veterans who are disabled or financially disadvantaged without regard to the patient's ability to pay. After adjustment for patient and hospital characteristics, blacks are 33% less likely than whites to receive cardiac catheterizations and 64% less likely to undergo any coronary revascularization procedure within 90 days of admission for an acute infarct.[116] These differences in procedure use are not limited to a single institution or state but are found in all regions of the nation.

The researchers offer several explanations for why blacks receive fewer cardiac procedures. First, blacks might have differences in disease severity, or symptoms and test results also may differ between black and whites. Second, racial differences in patient preference may exist—blacks may decline cardiac procedures when they are offered. Possibly whites are more assertive in pursuing cardiac interventions.

Finally, physicians may weigh the risks and benefits of interventional procedures differently for blacks and whites because there is belief that blacks have worse survival rates after coronary bypass surgery than whites. However, this has not been supported by multiple reviews of surgical outcomes.[117]

Finally, the researchers conclude that following AMI, blacks in the VHA had lower cardiac procedure uses which were not caused by differences in disease prevalence, contact with the medical community, or insurance coverage.

Wenneker and Epstein also ask why blacks undergo fewer cardiac procedures. They suggest that white patients might undergo more cardiac procedures because they are sicker than black patients and have a greater clinical need for intervention. Another possible explanation relates to the access issue, especially the ability to pay for needed medical care. A third explanation relates to socio-cultural differences between blacks and whites and their medical care preferences. The researchers speculate that these may be true interracial differences or may reflect differences between different socioeconomic classes because some studies have shown that blacks may be less likely to seek care or use health services even when they are available. Diehr and colleagues[118] note that blacks in Seattle are at least 10% less likely than whites to use health services offered by Blue Cross/Blue Shield, a health maintenance organization, or an independent practice association. There also is evidence from the Coronary Artery Surgery Study,[119] that whites may prefer a more technological approach for the treatment of coronary disease. Among subjects for whom a bypass was recommended, more than 90% of the whites agreed to surgery compared with only 81% of the blacks. Finally, interracial differences may reflect differences in care provided, perhaps unintentionally, on the basis of race. Previous studies have shown that African Americans undergoing surgery are more likely to receive care from a physician in training than from a senior staff surgeon.[120]

Kahn et al. undertook a study to examine the quality of care provided to insured, hospitalized Medicare patients who are black or poor as compared with those who are neither black nor poor. (Researchers combined black and poor subjects because the results for each group are similar.)

Using a nationally representative database of patients hospitalized with congestive heart failure, acute myocardial infarction (heart attack), pneumonia, and stroke, the researchers found differences in quality of care for acutely ill, elderly, insured patients who are black or poor as compared with others in similar hospitals. They say this effect is apparent across diseases and for each process measured. Black and poor patients also are more likely than other patients to be discharged with instability.[121]

Their research suggests that even among insured patients, those who are black or from poor neighborhoods receive worse care. The researchers indicated they do not know why insured Medicare patients who are black or poor experience lower quality of care and more instability at discharge than other patients cared for within the same hospital. They suggest that further research is needed "to clarify whether sociocultural and educational incongruity between providers and patients translated into misunderstandings about patients' preferences and expectation, and to evaluate the extent to which stereotyping, discrimination, or bias exist in the hospital setting."[122]

Although prior research has found that racial and poverty status influence access to care, the researchers report that racial characteristics and poverty status also influence the quality of care received by acutely ill, insured patients after they have gained access to the hospital.

AFRICAN AMERICAN HEALTH CARE SOLUTIONS

Sidel asks, "What is to be done?" He responds that "dealing effectively with these inner city problems is virtually impossible for doctors and other health workers, however well-informed and well-motivated they are, if they act alone. It is only through political action, by health workers acting together and in conjunction with others, that there is any hope of meeting these urgent needs."[123]

Although he foresees the need for a fundamental restructuring of a society in the long run, he thinks in the short run much can be done. "Those efforts usually lie more in the realm of the community, in 'public health' or 'social medicine,' rather than in the individual realm of 'preventive medicine,'" he writes. For example, he thinks responses such as restricting advertising of cigarettes and their easy availability that help entrap young people into the addiction of smoking are relatively easy compared to the development of programs for nutrition, housing, education, and public safety.

He also calls for community outreach programs to teach technical skills such as cardiopulmonary resuscitation and how to take blood pressures.

People can learn health education methods for work with their neighbors; and they can learn how to teach neighbors how to use the health care system more effectively, how to use preventive services, and how to organize the neighborhood for safety and for health.

Continued efforts to prevent unnecessary or untimely deaths will require evaluating both the social conditions that may cause disease as well as the factors that influence the efficacy of medical services. If it is agreed that mortality from these conditions is avoidable, then either health care services would be improved or the social conditions giving rise to these problems would be rectified.

Anderson et al. offers the following recommendations:

Involved target audience. Blacks should be involved in each stage of the planning and implementation of health care and education programs intended to be used primarily by black people.

Provide a service. Research institutions should avoid studying a minority patient populations without providing an appropriate and adequate service to the same community.

Empower people. Programs directed at improving the quality of life may focus on helping individuals change their behaviors and/or on influencing institutions to change their practices and policies toward a particular group.

Respect cultural diversity among blacks. Black people, although bound together by the experiences and effects of racism are still culturally diverse. Factors such as history, region, and community all play a role in this diversity. Educational and social programs must embrace and incorporate the cultural diversity of black people. They must seek to optimize the quality of life for African Americans while respecting their cultural beliefs, traditions, and lifestyles.[124]

The authors also point out that the black church has been identified as a means of promoting health issues and intervention programs and that the involvement of black church leaders is an important component in attracting community members and establishing rapport and credibility for the program with the community members. They say that black opinion leaders—teachers, preachers, nurses, social workers, and leaders of civic organizations—will lend credibility and visibility to health education efforts.[125]

Haywood says that two studies provide compelling evidence that intervention at the worksite can be an effective means of reducing overall risk of cardiovascular disease and of controlling hypertension in high-risk persons. However, evidence suggests that far more minorities employed are likely to be working in small businesses (with fewer than 20 employees), a fact that makes cost-effective screening programs and treatment programs harder to implement.

Haywood reports that one innovative approach to reach black males has been to carry out screening programs in local barber shops. He says to be most effective, education about the risks associated with high blood pressure should begin when education begins—at the grammar school level—and continue through high school. Education about risks of smoking, developing good eating habits, and the importance of early detection of high blood pressure are all part of developing good health habits.

Good public policy should dictate certain basic priorities and levels of funding for primary health care facilities that do not vary from election to election because changes in levels of funding can erode public confidence in the health care system and tend to confuse the very subpopulations most dependent upon public health care for medical attention.

Adler writes, "Whatever the solution, everyone agrees it will take time." He quotes Dionne Jones of the National Urban League in Washington, D.C.: "There is no one easy answer to this problem. We are going to have to involve more than government. We are going to have to bring to bear churches, parents, schools. We need to help parents instill values in their children. We need to revamp the education system."

CONCLUSIONS

The preceding information documents to a great extent the scope of the health care crisis facing African Americans, especially if they are poor and under-educated. However, little of the research has explored the attitudes of patients toward the health care system and their own view of health. There is much speculation about the role ethnic culture might play in barriers to seeking and using medical care. Most often, socioeconomic conditions are blamed for the discrepancy in health among different races in America. But, socioeconomic theories do not explain why poor whites and Hispanics are in better health than African Americans regardless of economic status. It seems logical that cultural norms and communication barriers may play a substantial role in the discrepancy.

Obviously, it is beyond the scope of this research to delve into public policy issues. The intent is to look more closely at attitudes regarding health care to determine if there are clearly definable African American attitudes that either allow them to screen out many or most health care messages or encourage them to avoid the health care system as much as possible. There is general agreement that better education programs—and thus, better ways to communicate with African Americans are needed.

Discrimination is another tantalizing element that is alluded to in some studies—all of which stop short of saying that health professionals allow their own prejudices to influence their treatment of black patients. Although there are some statistics that certainly support this theory, nothing appears in the literature about whether black patients themselves expect to be discriminated against in their local clinic, hospital, or doctor's office.

This study then will look next at communication theories that explain why African Americans might screen out media health care messages and, if this is the case, to suggest communication methods that might more effectively target people who need to focus on preventative measures (improved diet and exercise, screenings for preventable or treatable conditions, etc.). Possibly, more effective health care messages can be devised and channeled more efficiently to the target audience—African Americans. The second chapter will examine communication theories that might be used to better communicate with African Americans—particularly those who are poor and living in urban areas.

NOTES

1. Eugene Schwartz et al., "Black/White Comparisons of Deaths Preventable by Medical Intervention: United States and the District of Columbia 1980-1986, *International Journal of Epidemiology*, 19(3), 596.

2. Bureau of Census, *Current Population Survey*, (Washington, D.C.: U.S. Department of Commerce, 1987.) cited in Eugene Schwartz et al., "Black/White Comparisons of Deaths Preventable by Medical Intervention: United States and the District of Columbia 1980-1986, *International Journal of Epidemiology*, 19(3), 596.

3. National Center for Health Statistics, *Persons With and Without a Regular Source of Medical Care*. (Washington, D.C.: Series 10, No. 151, 1985.) cited in Schwartz et al., 596.

4. P. A. Butler, "Too Poor to Be Sick: Access to Medical Care for the Uninsured," *American Public Health Association*. (Washington, D.C.: 1988.) cited in Schwartz et al., 596.

5. Eric Adler, "Disease: Another Black Burden," *The Kansas City Star*, 24 July 1991, sec. A, p. 1.

6. Ibid.

7. Ibid.

8. Ibid., p.8.

9. Centers for Disease Control (U.S.: Atlanta, Ga., 1992).

10. Adler, sec. A, p. 8.

11. Missouri Department of Health, State Center for Health Statistics, *Missouri Vital Statistics 1988*. (Jefferson City): Missouri Department of Health, Division of Health Resources, State Center for Health Statistics, (1989).

12. Ross C. Brownson, James R. Davis, and Jian C. Chang, "Racial Differences in Cancer Mortality in Missouri," *Missouri Medicine,* (May, 1990): 291.

13. U.S. Public Health Service, *Cancer Among Blacks and Other Minorities: Statistical Profiles*. (Bethesda, MD): U.S. Department of Health and Human Services, Public Health Service, National Cancer Institute, NIH Publication No. 86-2785, (1986).

14. U.S. Public Health Service, *1987 Annual Cancer Statistics Review Including Cancer Trends: 1950-1985*. (Bethesda, MD): U.S. Department of Health and Human Services, Public Health Service, National Cancer Institute, NIH Publication No. 88-2789, (1988).

15. Brownson et al., p. 292.

16. U.S. Public Health Service, 1986.

17. Ibid.

18. Brownson et al., 293.

19. R. Doll and R. Peto, "The Causes of Cancer. Quantitative Estimates of Avoidable Risks of Cancer in the United States Today." *Journal of the National Cancer Institute* 66, (1981): 1191-1308.

20. U.S. Department of Health and Human Services, *Report of the Secretary's Task Force on Black & Minority Health. Volume III: Cancer*. (Washington D.C.): U.S. Government Printing Office, DHHS Publication No. 86-621-605, (1986).

21. Brownson et al., 293-294.

22. U.S. Department of Health and Human Services, *Report of the Secretary's Task Force on Black & Minority Health. Volume III: Cancer*. (Washington D.C.): U.S. Government Printing Office, DHHS Publication No. 86-621-605, (1986).

23. Brownson et al., 294.

24. Ibid.

25. Victor W. Sidel, "The Health of Poor and Minority People in the Inner City," *New York State Journal of Medicine*, Vol. 91 No. 5, (May 1991), 180.

26. Ibid., 181.

27. Ibid.

28. Marcia K. Petchers and Sharon E. Milligan, "Access to Health Care in a Black Urban Elderly Populations," *Gerontologist*, Vol. 28 No. 2, (April 1988): 214.

29. J. Gylys and B. Gylys, "Cultural Influences and the Medical Behavior of Low Income Groups," *Journal of the National Medical Association*, 66, (1974): 310-313.

30. Petchers and Milligan, 216.

31. Robert M. Anderson et al., "Barriers to Improving Diabetes Care for Blacks," *Diabetes Care*, Vol. 14, No. 7, (July 1991): 605.

32. Ibid., 606.

33. Ibid.

34. S. Hopper, "Diabetes as a Stigmatized Condition: the Case of Low-Income Patients in the United States," *Social Science Medicine*, 15B, (1981): 11-19.

35. Anderson et al., 606.

36. A. R. VanSon, "Crossing Cultural and Economic Boundaries," In *Diabetes and Patient Education: A Daily Nursing Challenge* (New York: Appleton-Century-Crofts, 1981), 160-177.

37. S. Hopper, "Meeting the Needs of the Economically Deprived Diabetic," *Nurse Clinician of North America*, 18, (1983): 813-825, cited in Anderson et al., 606.

38. VanSon, 160-177, cited in Anderson et al., 606.

39. Anderson, 606.

40. Ibid., 606-607.

41. Ibid., 607.

42. Robert J. Blendon et al., "Access to Medical Care for Black and White Americans A Matter of Continuing Concern," *Journal of the American Medical Association*, Vol. 261, No. 2, (1989): 278.

43. National Center for Health Statistics, *Health, United States, 1987*, DHHS Publication (PHS) 88-1232. (Washington, D.C.): Department of Health and Human Services, (1987).

44. Blendon et al., 279.

45. Ibid., 279.

46. Ibid., 280.

47. K. Erdman and S. Wolfe, *"Poor Health Care for Poor Americans: A Ranking of State Medicaid Programs,"* (Washington D.C.): Public Citizen Health Research Group, (1987), cited in Blendon et al., 280.

48. Blendon et al., 280.

49. Ibid., 280.

50. Ibid., 280-281.

51. *Access to Health Care in the United States: Results of a 1986 Survey—Special Report No. 2.* (Princeton, NJ): Robert Wood Johnson Foundation, (1987).

52. *Health Status of the Disadvantaged—Chartbook 1986. United States.* U.S. Department of Health and Human Services (DHHS) Publication No. HRS-P-DV86-2. (Washington, D.C.): Health Resources and Services Administration, (1986).

53. Paula Braveman et al., "Women and Medicine: Women Without Health Insurance Links Between Access, Poverty, Ethnicity, and Health," *Western Journal of Medicine*, December (1988): 709.

54. Public Health Service Task Force on Women's Issues: *Women's Health Report*, 100, (Washington, D.C.): Department of Public Health, (1985): 73-105, cited in Braveman et al., 709.

55. *Health Status of Minorities and Low-Income Groups*, U.S. Department of Health, Education and Welfare (DHEW) publication No. HRA 790627. (Washington, D.C.): Health Resources Administration, (1978) cited in Braveman et al., 709.

56. *Health United States 1984*, US DHHS Publication No. (PHS)85-1232. (Hyattsville, Md.): National Center for Health Statistics, (1984) cited in Braveman et al., 709.

57. Ibid.

58. Braveman et al., 709.

59. Shelly I. White-Means and Michael C. Thornton, "Nonemergency Visits to Hospital Emergency Rooms: A Comparison of Blacks and Whites," *The Milbank Quarterly*, Vol 67, No. 1, (1989): 35.

60. Ibid.

61. Ibid., 36.

62. Ibid., 50.

63. Ibid., 51.

64. Ibid., 52.

65. *Report of the Secretary's Task Force on Black Minority Health, VI: Infant Mortality and Low Birthweight.* (Washington, DC): U.S. Department of Health and Human Services, (1986).

66. Christiane B. Hale, and Charlotte M. Druschel, "Infant Mortality Among Moderately Low Birth Weight Infants in Alabama, 1980 to 1983," *Pediatrics*, Vol. 84 No. 2, (August 1989): 285.

67. Ibid., 289.

68. Anne Scupholme, Euan G. Robertson, and A. Susan Kamons, "Barriers to Prenatal Care in a Multiethnic, Urban Sample," *Journal of Nurse-Midwifery*, Vol. 36 No. 2, (March/April, 1991): 111.

69. Ibid.

70. Ibid., 114.

71. *U.S. Department of Health and Human Resources: Health 1987.* (Bethesda, MD): U.S. Government Printing Office, (1987) cited in Scupholme et al., 115.

72. Scupholme, 115.

73. Ibid., 116.

74. Ibid.

75. National Diabetes Data Group, *Diabetes in America*, (Bethesda, MD): Department of Health and Human Services, NIH publication No. 85-1468 (1985).

76. American Diabetes Association, *Diabetes: An Equal Opportunity Disease*, (Alexandria, VA): Diabetes Information Service Center, (1989).

77. Anderson et al., 605.

78. Ibid.

79. Ibid.

80. Ibid.

81. Ibid., 607.

82. Ibid., 154.

83. Ibid.

84. Edgar J. Kenton, "Access to Neurological Care for Minorities," *Archives of Neurology*, 48, (May 1991): 480.

85. Robert Wood Johnson Foundation Special Report, *Access to Health Care in the United States: Results of a 1986 Survey,* (Princeton, NJ): Robert Wood Johnson Foundation, (1987), cited in Kenton, 480.

86. National Center for Health Statistics, *Vital Statistics of the United States, 1979: Mortality,* (Washington, D.C.): Public Health Service, 2 pt A, (1984): U.S. Department of Health and Human Services Publication (PHS)84-1101 cited in Kenton, 480.

87. Kenton, 481.

88. Ibid., 480.

89. Ibid., 481.

90. L. Julian Haywood, "Hypertension in Minority Populations," *The American Journal of Medicine*, 88 (suppl 3B), (March 12, 1990), 17s.

91. Ibid., 18s.

92. Catherine C. Boring, Teresa S. Squires and Clark W. Heath, Jr., "Cancer Statistics for African Americans," *CA—A Cancer Journal for Clinicians*, 41, (May/June 1991): 7.

93. L.A.G. Ries , B.F. Hankey, B.K. Edwards, *Cancer Statistics Review 1973-1988,*. NIH Publication No 91-2789, (Bethesda, MD): National Cancer Institute, (1991) cited in Boring et al., 7 .

94. Boring et al., 14.

95. Mayer and McWhorter, 773.

96. R.F. Gillum, "Coronary Heart Disease in Black Populations I: Mortality and Morbidity," *American Heart Journal*, 104, (1982): 839-851 cited in David S. Strogatz, "Use of Medical Care for Chest Pain: Differences between Blacks and Whites," *American Journal of Public Health*, Vol. 80 No. 3, (March 1990): 290.

97. M.J. Henderson and D.D. Savage, "Prevalence and Incidence of Ischemic Heart Disease in United States' Black and White Populations," *Report of the Secretary's Task Force on Black and Minority Health IV Cardiovascular and Cerebrovascular Disease,* (Washington, D.C.): Government Printing Office, (1986): 620-638 cited in Strogatz, 290.

98. A.B. Weisse, P.D. Abiuso, and I.S. Thind, "Acute Myocardial Infarction in Newark, NJ," *Archives of Internal Medicine,* 137, (1977): 1402-1405, cited in Strogatz, 290.

99. J.E. Keil, D.E. Saunders, D.T. Lackland, et al., "Acute Myocardial Infarction: Period Prevalence, Case Fatality and Comparison of Black and White Cases in Urban and Rural Areas of South Carolina," *America Heart Journal,* 109, (1985): 776-784, cited in Strogatz, 290.

100. David S. Strogatz, "Use of Medical Care for Chest Pain: Differences between Blacks and Whites," *American Journal of Public Health*, Vol. 80 No. 3, (March 1990): 290.

101. Ibid.

102. E. Berkanovic and C. Telesky, "Mexican-American, Black-American and White- American Differences in Reporting Illnesses, Disability and Physician Visits for Illnesses," *Social Science in Medicine*, 20, (1985): 567-577, cited in Strogatz, 292.

103. Strogatz, 292-293.

104. Ibid., 293.

105. Joel S. Weissman et al., "Delayed Access to: Risk Factors, Reasons, and Consequences," *Annals of Internal Medicine*, Vol. 114 No. 4, (Feb. 15, 1991): 325.

106. Ibid.

107. Ibid.

108. Ibid., 329.

109. Council Report, *Black-White Disparities in Health Care,* (Chicago, IL): Council on Ethical and Judicial Affairs, American Medical Association (1989), 2344.

110. Ibid., 2345.

111. J. Yergan et al., "Relationship Between Patient Race and the Intensity of Hospital Services," *Medical Care,* 25, (1987): 592-603, cited in Council Report, 2345.

112. Council Report, 2344.

113. Ibid., 2345.

114. Ibid., 2345.

115. Ibid.

116. Eric D. Peterson et al., "Racial Variation in Cardiac Procedure Use and Survival Following Acute Myocardial Infarction in the Department of Veterans Affairs," *Journal of the American Medical Association,* Vol. 271 No. 15, (April 20, 1994): 1178.

117. Ibid., 1179.

118. P. Diehr, D.P. Martin, K.F. Price et al., "Use of Ambulatory Care Services in Three Provider Plans," *American Journal of Public Health,* 74, (1984): 47-51, cited in Mark B. Wenneker and Arnold M. Epstein, "Racial Inequalities in the Use of Procedures for Patients With Ischemic Heart Disease in Massachusetts," *Journal of the American Medical Association,* Vol. 261 No. 2, (Jan. 13, 1989): 256.

119. C. Maynard, L.D. Fisher, E.R. Passamani et al., "Blacks in the Coronary Artery Surgery Study," *Circulation,* 74, (1986): 64-71 cited in Wenneker and Epstein, 256.

120. L.D. Egbert and I.L. Rothman, "Relation Between Race and Economic Status of Patients and Who Performs Their Surgery," *New England Journal of Medicine,* 297, (1977): 90-91.

121. Katherine L. Kahn, Marjorie L. Pearson, Ellen R. Harrison et al., "Healthcare for Black and Poor Hospitalized Medicare Patients," *Journal of the American Medical Association,* Vol. 271 No. 15, (April 20, 1994): 1172.

122. Ibid., 1173.

123. Sidel, 181.

124. Anderson et al., 607.

125. Ibid.

CHAPTER III

Communication Theories Relevant to Health Care Professionals

Health care professionals and public relations/marketing specialists who are attempting to introduce new treatments or who want to encourage changes in lifestyle need to be aware of some communication theories. Mass communication theory is of particular importance because much of the communication that is taking place today involves mass media channels (television, radio, newspapers, magazines and the Internet). For example, who can dispute that asprin commercials are a major source of information about pain relief and recovery from heart attacks? The Internet has become a source of information and disinformation about many diseases and treatments. For example, there are now discussion groups devoted to people afflicted with the same disease, but there are also many World Wide Web sites devoted to selling "cures" that have never been scientifically proven or FDA approved.

Physicians should be aware of the various ways patients get and assimilate information. That often involves, at the very least, some knowledge of mass communication channels and the way people communicate—particularly ethnic or economic minorities that have developed their own system of communicating about health care and "cures."

Although there has been much written about the processes of communication and about the role of the audience in mass communication, little has been proven about whether mass communication actually has an effect on individual or group *behavior*. Part of the difficulty, of course, is being able to measure behavior change. The next best alternative is to examine attitudes and to accept some basic assumptions that if attitudes change, behaviors could change as well.

DeFleur and Ball-Rokeach say that the members of contemporary urban-industrial societies are not all similar. They can be conceptually arranged into well-defined social categories insofar as they shared some common characteristics, such as social class, religion, ethnic identity, rural-urban residence, and so on.[1] However, studies have begun to show that people in any particular grouping, such as young urban professionals or African Americans, have many similarities that have a significant impact on their behavior. Researchers discovered that within such categories people shared a somewhat distinctive way of life that made up a kind of "microculture" distinct from that of the larger society.[2] Examples of this are specialized language (dialect, idioms, slang, etc.), distinctive attitudes (such as the concept of machoism among Hispanics), values, beliefs, and skills related to their positions and activities in the social structure (such as religion, family structure, and social clubs or organizations). These subgroups also could have problems that are not shared by society at large (such as discrimination, health problems, housing, etc.).

It is beyond the scope of this research to measure changes in behaviors. Rather, the focus is on identifying attitudes and then suggesting possible health campaign strategies that might first reach the target audience and then make changes in the attitudes of some audience members. This in turn could lead to behavior changes.

DeFleur and Ball-Rokeach list five major perspectives of human communication:

1. Communication is a *semantic* process; it is dependent upon symbols and rules for their use that have been selected by a given language community.
2. It is a *neurobiological* process in which meanings for particular symbols are recorded in the memory functions of individuals. Thus, the central nervous system plays a key role in the storage and recovery of internal meaning experiences.
3. It is a *psychological* process; the meanings of words or other symbols to a given individual are acquired through *learning*. Such meanings play a central part in perceiving the world and responding to it.

4. Human communication is a *cultural* process; language is a set of cultural conventions. That is, the language of any society is a set of postures, gestures, symbols, and their arrangements that have shared or agreed-upon interpretations.

5. Communication is a *social* process; it is the principal means by which human beings are able to *interact* in meaningful ways. Thus, through symbolic interchange, human beings can play roles, understand the norms of a group, apply social sanctions, and appraise each other's actions within a system of shared values. This integration of perspectives shows once again how indispensable communication is to human beings.[3]

This study focuses primarily on cultural processes (the differences in the way African Americans compared to others in American society view health care and health care messages) and social processes (whether friends, family members, and doctors are more credible than mass media).

CONTEMPORARY THEORIES OF MASS COMMUNICATION

Modern communication assumes that people are active—rather than passive—receivers of information. Psychologists find individual differences in people's needs, attitudes, values, and other personality variables. Lowery and DeFleur have proposed a new theory that they refer to as the *theory of selective influence* based on individual differences.[4] They summarize its basic ideas as follows:

1. The media present messages to the members of mass society, but those messages are received and interpreted selectively.

2. The basis of this selectivity lies in variations in habits of perception among members of the society.

3. Variations in habits of perception occur because each individual has a unique personal organization of beliefs, attitudes, values, needs, and modes of experiencing gratification that has been acquired through learning.

4. Because perception is selective, interpretation, retention and response to media messages are also selective and variable.

5. Thus, the effects of the media are neither uniform, powerful, nor direct. Their influences are selective and limited by individual psychological differences.[5]

DeFleur and Ball-Rokeach say the logical implication of this theory is that "persuasive messages should be tailored to those with specific interests, needs, values, beliefs, and the like. This segmented approach was more likely to achieve the desired goals than the 'one message fits all' approach."[6] Before a persuasive campaign is designed, the specific cognitive characteristics of the target audiences have to be identified. To make the message more effective, appeals, arguments, slogans, and other features can be included in the content to attract the attention of the target audience in an attempt to trigger the desired behavior.

DeFleur and Ball-Rokeach attribute this theory to laying the groundwork "for the concept of market segmentation as a principle for understanding and developing strategies to sell goods, politicians, and pro-social behavior among large media audiences." This approach "emphasized the need for market research aimed at identifying what kinds of people bought, voted, gave, or otherwise acted on the basis of what motivations, interests, attitudes, or other psychological conditions" and that "research into the 'psycho-dynamics' of persuasion used in advertising, public information campaigns, and marketing brought the methodology of psychological experimentation and measurement to market research." Measuring psychological variables (such as preferences, attitudes, needs, and values) provides insight into consumer and voter motivations.[7] Before effective health messages can be transmitted, it is important to identify attitudes toward the health care system and toward health care providers.

Davison et al. suggest "the most important conclusion to be drawn from research on the effects of mass media on information level is that there is no direct relationship between exposure to information and learning of information."[8] The question, they say, is not whether mass communications could or could not affect attitudes, but rather under what conditions there would be an effect and under what conditions no effect or very little effect.[9]

Four characteristics of audiences seem to be particularly important in accounting for different attitudinal effects, according to Davison et al.:

First, there are personality and educational differences. . . . Second, people are situated in a variety of social settings. . . . Third, the attitudes that any one person has may vary in strength. . . . Fourth, external events may affect audience attitudes.[10]

They argue that the media can actually change or form new attitudes, or they can reinforce or activate existing attitudes.[11] For example, they say it seems reasonable to assume that the civil rights and women's rights movements would have developed more slowly if they had not received so much attention in mass communications, but there is no way to know whether these movements might not have developed anyway. "Perhaps the media activated and reinforced existing attitudes to a point where they led to actions that advanced these movements, for example, demonstrations, the passage of legislation, and changes in employment policies," they say.[12] Different types of people in an audience selected and interpreted mass communication content in widely variant ways.[13]

Regarding the basic principles of selectivity, Davison et al. say the most important ones include:

Consistency. We have a tendency to favor communications that are congruent with our existing ideas over information that conflicts with our mental map of the world.

Utility. We select communications that we think will be helpful in satisfying some need or that will give us pleasure.

Availability. If we have no preference for one communication over another, we will expose ourselves to the one that is more easily available.[14]

They argue that all of these principles should be taken into account by any practitioner of mass communication who is seeking to gain the attention of a particular audience.[15]

The most effective health messages aimed at African Americans, therefore, should not conflict with their reality, should satisfy some need they have, and should be distributed through the communication channels that are most pervasive in African American communities.

DeFleur and Ball-Rokeach discuss four basic principles that they say influence the way audiences attend to the media, interpret what they are exposed to, remember media content, and are thereby influenced in their actions. These principles are concerned with selective attention, perception, recall, and action, and they lie at the heart of the selective influence theories:

1. *The principle of selective attention.* There are so many competing messages that people cannot possibly attend to everything that is directed toward them without suffering "instant overload." People, therefore, develop "mental filters" that screen out vast amounts of information.[16]

2. *The principle of selective perception.* Because of differences in interests, beliefs, prior knowledge, attitudes, needs, and values, individuals will perceive or attribute meaning to virtually any complex stimulus differently than will people with different cognitive structures. For example, that African Americans "often interpret news stories about capital punishment, busing, school dropouts, and other social issues that have an impact on black people in ways that are not the same as the interpretations of whites."[17] It is likely that they interpret health messages differently as well. Values, needs, beliefs, and attitudes, then, should be studied before formulating health messages.

3. *The principle of selective recall.* Some kinds of content for some kinds of people will be actively remembered for a long time, while others with different cognitive structures, category memberships, and social linkages may forget the same material quickly.[18]

4. *The principle of selective action.* Not everyone acts in the same way as a result of being exposed to the same media message. Before action can take place, an individual (member of an audience) has to attend to the media presentation, perceive its meaning, and remember its content.[19]

Davison et al. pointed to selectivity's role in learning:

> Theories that attempt to explain selectivity are helpful in accounting for the substantial learning from the mass media in some cases and the seeming absence of learning in others. If people want information, for whatever reasons, they are likely to learn. If they don't want information, they are unlikely to absorb it. When they don't care one way or the other, but are exposed to mass media, they will learn some things anyway.[20]

They concluded that "those who regularly expose themselves to the news media are better informed than those who do not."[21] This theory suggests that there are conditions under which the majority of African Americans will selectively avoid health messages. For example, they may automatically pay less attention to messages that feature white people than ones that include or feature African Americans.

SOCIAL CATEGORIES THEORY

Lowery and DeFleur report that "as the selective nature of human perception was being realized by media researchers, another form of selective influence was found. This was what sociologists call *social categories*." People in different positions in the social structure act differently, including their mass communication behavior. The rich and the poor, males and females, the educated and the uneducated, for example, represent distinctive categories of people in the complex social system. Lowery and DeFleur emphasize that the behavior *within any category* tends to be remarkably similar. They give as examples young, affluent females with reasonably high education level who read *Vogue*, *Glamour* and similar magazines and poor, black, male youths living in the inner city who read comic books but not the editorial section of the newspaper. They call this the *theory of selectivity based on social categories*.[22] The theory can be summarized in these terms:

1. The media present messages to the members of the mass society but they are received and interpreted selectively.
2. An important basis of this selectivity lies in the location of the individual in the differentiated social structure.
3. That social structure is composed of numerous categories of people, defined by such factors as age, sex, income, education, and occupation.
4. Patterns of media attention and response are shaped by the factors that define these categories, making response to mass communication somewhat similar in each.
5. Thus, the effects of the media are neither uniform, powerful, nor direct, but are selective and limited by social category influences.[23]

It can be expected, therefore, that once people are "factored" into categories, their behavior can be predicted and messages can be targeted more effectively.

"DEMOGRAPHICS" AS A BASIS OF MARKET SEGMENTATION

DeFleur and Ball-Rokeach emphasized that the study of social categories (groups of people with specific characteristics and behaviors) led to the development of market segmentation. This development, in turn, required the survey research techniques "to study the clusters of predispositions, preferences, and other aspects of consumer or voter behavior as these differed among differential kinds of people." They say research shows that there are significant differences between the purchasing habits and consuming behavior of people of different incomes, ages, levels of education, ethnic backgrounds, and so on.[24] The recent Sears Foundation/National Newspaper Publishers Association survey of African Americans to determine media and buying habits is a good example. Several demographic variables were included to determine if the African American market can be segmented into definable groups based on income, education, gender, etc.[25] This book also is concerned with demographics and whether they can help describe various groups of people classified by attitudes.

PERSUASION THEORY INVOLVING ATTITUDES AND OPINIONS

Hovland and his associates studied attitudes and opinion change in order to determine how persuasion occurs. Lowery and DeFleur say they viewed attitudes and opinions as intimately related, yet analytically distinct. The term "opinion" refers to "interpretations, expectations, and evaluations," which could include "beliefs about the intentions of others, anticipations of future events, or appraisals of the consequences of alternate courses of action." "Attitude," on the other hand, refers to "explicit responses approaching or avoiding some object, person, group, or symbol."[26]

Hovland and his associates believed that three variables are important in the learning of new attitudes: attention, comprehension, and acceptance:

The first of these factors, *attention*, recognizes the fact that not all message stimuli that a person encounters are noticed. . . . The second factor posited by Hovland and his colleagues, *comprehension*, recognizes the fact that some messages may be too complex and too ambiguous for their intended audience to understand. . . . Finally, a person must decide to accept the communication before any real attitude change takes place. The degree of acceptance is largely related to the incentives that are offered.[27]

Lowery and DeFleur summarize Hovland's theoretical model of changing attitudes or opinions in this way:

1. A recommended opinion (the stimulus) is presented.
2. Assuming that the subjects have paid attention to and understood the message, the audience responds or reacts. That is, they think about their initial opinions and also about the recommended opinion.
3. The subjects will change their attitudes if incentives (rewards) for making a new response are greater than the incentives for making the old response.[28]

Health care messages must first be presented in an interesting or dramatic way to attract attention. The literacy level of the target audience must be considered so that messages are not too complicated or too patronizing. Some sort of incentive should be offered for behavior change. Then, the audience must be evaluated to determine whether changes in attitudes and behaviors have occurred.

Hovland and his associates argue that individuals' conforming tendencies stem from membership in groups based on knowledge of what behavior is expected of them by other members and on the individual's motivation to live up to those expectations. Group norms, therefore, tend to make the individual resistant to change and can interfere with the effectiveness of persuasive communications. This hypothesis leads to interest in "counter-norm communications," messages that argue in direct opposition to group norms.[29]

Lowery and DeFleur say research has shown that the more highly persons value membership in a group, the more closely their attitudes and opinion conformed to the consensus within that group.[30] Kelley and Volkhart hypothesized that individuals who highly value their membership in a group will be less influenced by communications contrary to the group's norms than will those who do not value membership as much. That is, opinion change will be inversely related to the degree to which the person values group membership.[31] Someone who takes pride in being a member of an African American community may identify more with messages that evoke feelings of membership than those who have distanced themselves from the community.

The effects of a communication may partly depend on the characteristics of individual members of the audience. Hovland et al. believe that investigating personality factors could lead to predictions about the way in which an individual or groups of individuals might respond. They thought it possible to predict the degree to which a persuasive communication will succeed in changing beliefs and attitudes.[32]

Hovland and his associates investigated two general types of personality factors: "intellectual abilities" and "motive factors." Intellectual abilities refer to the way an individual attends to, interprets, and assimilates the many communications to which he or she is constantly exposed. Motive factors refer to predominant personality needs, emotional disturbances, defense mechanisms, frustration tolerance, thresholds of excitability, etc., which may facilitate or interfere with a person's responsiveness to many different types of persuasive communications.

The authors found a complex relationship between intellectual ability and persuasibility. They found it is easier to persuade individuals with high intelligence than those low in intellectual ability because "the former have more ability to draw valid inferences when exposed to persuasive communications that rely primarily on impressive logical arguments" even though they also are more likely to be critical of the arguments presented.[33] Individuals with high intelligence, then, are less likely to be influenced "when they are exposed to persuasive communications which rely primarily on unsupported generalities or upon false, illogical, irrelevant argumentation."[34] This would suggest that different types of communication messages might have to be devised to reach those who are literate and well-educated than for those that function at a low intellectual level. For example, information about infant and child care might need to be cast in different forms for a 30-year-old career woman versus a teen-age mother who drops out of high school.

MODELING THEORY

Lowery and DeFleur say a new theoretical formulation came from psychology as an adaptation of social learning theory. The psychological theory showed how exposure to modeled behavior in mass communication content "could provide the individual with a learning source for the adoption of forms of action that could become a more or less permanent part of the person's mode of coping with recurring problems." This formulation has come to be called modeling theory and can be summarized as follows:

1. The individual perceives a form of behavior described or portrayed by a character in media content.
2. The individual judges this behavior to be attractive and potentially useful for coping with some personal situation that has arisen or might arise.
3. The portrayed behavior is reproduced by the individual in a relevant personal situation.
4. The reproduced behavior proves useful or effective in coping with the situation, thereby rewarding the individual.
5. With further use, the modeled behavior becomes the person's habitual way of handling that type of situation, unless it is no longer effective and rewarding.[35]

Lowery and DeFleur point out that the important idea is that the theory does not assume that people see some action in media content and then immediately and uniformly imitate that action; but modeling may come later and new behaviors may slowly become a part of the person's repertoire, depending upon the frequency of relevant occasions for its use. In a population, at least some people might be influenced indirectly over a long period of time by media-modeled behaviors.[36] This idea is at least partly responsible for the ban on cigarette advertising and the reduction of showing people smoking on television and the restrictions placed on advertisements of alcoholic beverages.

This theory seems to argue for long-term health care campaigns with as much media saturation as possible. For example, if people are shown how to eat a low-fat diet often enough and over a long enough period of time, they may begin to purchase food lower in fat. Also, if women are shown enough information about how to do self-breast examinations, they may start doing the checks on a regular basis. Enlisting the cooperation of entertainment and sports personalities as spokespersons may also be effective.

MEANING THEORY

Lowery and DeFleur's second new theoretical formulation came from sociology and anthropology as an adaptation of theories concerning the nature of symbolic interaction and the influence of language on behavior. Regarding this theory, Lowery and DeFleur say, "From anthropology came the conclusion that the language used by a given people had a profound influence on the manner in which they perceived, experienced, and acted upon the physical and social worlds around them." They summarize the principal propositions of *meaning theory* as follows:

1. The individual perceives a situation described or portrayed in media content.
2. That situation is labelled by a standardized symbol or symbols from the shared language.
3. The media content effectively links the label and the portrayed meaning for the individual.
4. By such presentations, the media can establish new meanings, extend older ones to include new elements, substitute alternative meaning for older ones, or stabilize the language conventions concerning the shared meaning for symbols in the language community.
5. Since language (standardized labels and their shared meanings) is a critical factor shaping perception, interpretation, and decision concerning action, the media can have powerful, indirect and long-term effects.[37]

Lowery and DeFleur conclude that "a medium like television can show us how to interpret such labels as 'women,' 'black people,' 'sexual attractiveness,' and a host of other terms." They speculate that the influence of the media is probably indirect and long-term. There also is an African American "language" which often is viewed as "incorrect speech." However, using this language for some health messages could be appropriate and effective. Meaning theory suggests that to communicate with African

Americans it is important to understand the language they use (slang, idioms, etc.) and to select carefully words used in health care messages that can be easily understood and not misconstrued.

CONSISTENCY THEORIES

Davison et al. contend individuals consciously or subconsciously select from the flow of communications those ideas that fit in with their attitudes and values and that are consistent with their existing beliefs about the world. At the same time, individuals ignore, dismiss, misunderstand, or forget those communications that would be "dissonant"—that would not fit in.[38] For example, an African American who believes in home remedies for the care of arthritis would not be likely to read an article about surgery options or might not absorb much information if he or she did read it. On the other hand, someone who is eligible for Medicare might purchase a newspaper or magazine featuring a story about Congressional revisions in Medicare benefits and eligibility.

The authors group together three principal theories—known as the theories of balance, congruity, and dissonance.[39] The point out that a mechanism people use to maintain and strengthen their existing view of the world and avoid having it disturbed by incongruent or unbalancing information, is *selective exposure*. People will expose themselves to messages that are consistent with their attitudes and beliefs while avoiding other messages or paying attention only to certain parts of the communication and disregarding the rest.[40] Social scientists usually refer to this as *selective perception*. If people do have to pay attention to a potentially disturbing message, they may interpret it so that it will not conflict with existing ideas. For example, someone who smokes who is exposed to an anti-smoking message in his or her doctor's waiting room might conclude that the message is untrue or for one reason or another does not apply to him or her. Davison et al. calls this behavior *selective interpretation*.[41] Finally, people may forget dissonant information or may remember it in distorted form, a behavior known as *selective recall*. For example, if African American smokers were asked later about the content of the anti-smoking message, they may not recall statistics about African Americans, or they may say the information applied only to whites.

The authors reported the results of research conducted when the mini-series "Roots" was broadcast in 1977:

> Black viewers were found to regard the series as more accurate historically than did whites. They also were more likely than whites to feel that the drama's portrayal of white and black roles was reasonably true to life. Most white viewers seem to have been able to interpret the story in such a way that it did not disturb their existing attitudes and beliefs. It may have had a greater impact on attitudes among blacks, but the researchers were unable to find enough blacks who had *not* viewed the series to compare their attitudes with the attitudes of those who had seen it.[42]

MEDIA SYSTEM DEPENDENCY THEORY

The media system dependency theory, related to consistency theories, involves *active selectors* and *casual observers*. DeFleur and Ball-Rokeach contend that *active selectors* will expose themselves to "media content that they have reason to expect will help them to achieve one or more of their understanding, orientations, or play goals."[43] Their expectations are based upon (1) their prior experience, (2) conversation with their interpersonal associates (friends and co-workers), or (3) cues obtained from media sources (advertising or reviews).

Casual observers, DeFleur and Ball-Rokeach say, "encounter media content incidentally with no preformed expectations (e.g., walking into a laundromat where the TV is on)." When exposure occurs, some may find that one or more dependency is activated that motivates them to continue exposure, while others may not experience dependency activation and might terminate exposure when the situation permits. They argue that where the content is not connecting with the individual's motivations, continued exposure would be due to situational demands. Most people are active selectors much of the time and casual observers some of the time.[44]

The second step in this process has to do with different intensities in exposure and dependency. DeFleur and Ball-Rokeach say, "Not all people who selectively expose themselves to certain media content will do so with the same degree of dependency, nor will all people who have their dependencies activated during incidental exposure." They concluded that variations in intensity of individuals' media dependencies will be a function of differences in:

1. Personal goals.
2. Personal and social environments.
3. Expectations with regard to the potential utility of the specific media content under consideration.
4. Ease of access to that content.[45]

DeFleur and Ball-Rokeach say an example of how variations in people's personal and social environs affect the intensity of dependency concerns serious health problems. "People who are, themselves, or who have loved ones who are seriously ill often develop strong media dependencies in order to gain access to relevant information that might contribute to their finding the best medical and support services. They should, for example, be particularly responsive to relevant health information presented in talk shows, dramas, health news columns, and the like," they say. Access to media information resources is often necessary to the resolution of ambiguity and the reduction of real or potential threat.

DeFleur and Ball-Rokeach say they can hypothesize that "the greater the intensity of relevant media dependencies, the greater the degree of (1) cognitive arousal (catching and maintaining people's attention) and (2) affective arousal (arousing their emotions)."

The third step in this process is *involvement,* which refers to more than arousal; it refers to active participation in information processing. DeFleur and Ball-Rokeach's hypothesis is that "people who have been cognitively and affectively aroused will engage in the kind of careful processing of information that will allow them to recall or remember the information after exposure." They say, "Research suggests that high involvement is a particularly important consideration in successful public health media campaigns designed to get audiences to change their beliefs or behavior, such as to stop smoking, start exercising, or get medical checkups."[46]

The final step in the media system dependency effects process is that "individuals who have become intensely involved in information processing are more likely to be affected by their exposure to media content." DeFleur and Ball-Rokeach doubt that *cognitive* effects, or effects on perceptions, attitudes, knowledge, or values can be separated from *affective* effects, such as feelings of fear, happiness, sentiment, or hatred.[47] They argue that most attitude changes carry with them some change of liking or disliking of an object or situation. Effects on behavior are another story. DeFleur and Ball-Rokeach say there has been a tendency to abandon efforts to demonstrate media effects on behavior mainly because attempts to show that attitude change produces change in behavior have been disappointing.[48]

USES AND GRATIFICATIONS

Lowery and DeFleur consider uses and gratifications theory to be a psychological approach that focuses on the *individual* and is concerned with the conative, cognitive, and affective organizations.[49] Psychologists, according to Lowery and DeFleur, attempt to get inside the head to "search for variables and generalizations that can explain what motivates individuals to act, what leads a person to behave in new ways, and what maintains patterns of responses already established."[50]

Davison et al. say that according to the uses and gratifications approach (sometimes referred to as utility theory) individuals pay attention to, perceive, and remember information that is pleasurable or that will in some way help to satisfy their needs or interests. Individuals will attend to information they expect to be useful or to give satisfaction regardless of whether it is in accord with their existing ideas (according to Katz, Blumler, and Gurevitch, 1974).[51]

Newspapers have long "rewarded" people by providing a variety of information and providing headlines that help people select what they want to read and leads that often distill the basic ideas of a story quickly. Television, of course, provides both "entertainment" programming and "news" programming. Stephenson would likely argue that even "news" programming can be entertaining. He suggested mass communications are a form of "play" in American society, providing the kinds of gratifications that the term implies.[52]

Katz, Blumler, and Gurevitch listed five elements they consider important in understanding the uses and gratifications model:

1. The audience is conceived of as active, that is, an important part of mass media use is assumed to be goal directed (McQuail, Blumler and Brown, 1972).

2. In the mass communication process much initiative in linking need gratification and media choice lies with the audience member.
3. The media compete with other sources of need satisfaction.
4. Methodologically speaking, many of the goals of mass media use can be derived from data supplied by individual audience members themselves.
5. Value judgments about the cultural significance of mass communications shouldbe suspended while audience orientations are explored on their own

Blumler and Katz described the uses and gratifications approach as one concerned with the nature and origins of people's needs that play a part in leading them to different patterns of media exposure. Lowery and DeFleur say the Blumler and Katz approach offers the following policy implications:

> If the form of content that satisfies the needs of a particular segment of the audience (e.g., middle-class housewives, the elderly, single males, blacks, and so on) can be identified, media presentations incorporating that content can be used to capture and hold the attention of such segments. If the content gratifies their needs, such presentations would appear to be dependable vehicles for the presentation of advertising messages, political campaigns, or other appeals. In this sense, needs gratifications research is relevant to the use of the media for deliberate persuasion.[53]

Although several studies have attempted to list the needs satisfied by media content, or typologies of motivations and functions involved in attention to mass communication, Davison et al. say no agreement exists as to why people select particular content, what needs a given form of content satisfies, or how such gratification leads to behavioral consequences.[54]

Although "needs" have been categorized in various ways, Katz, Gurevitch, and Haas list the following:

> *Cognitive needs,* having to do with acquiring information, knowledge, and understanding.
> *Affective needs,* having to do with emotional or aesthetic experiences, including the need for love and friendship, the desire to see beautiful things.
> *Personal integrative needs,* for confidence, stability, status, reassurance.

Social integrative needs, for strengthening contacts with family, friends, and other people in general.
Tension-release needs, for escape and diversion.[55]

According to utility theory, if individuals expect a communication to be uninteresting or unpleasant, they probably will disregard or forget it or avoid exposure altogether. Smokers, for example, might leave the room or turn their attention to something else if a television news broadcast runs a story about the health risks associated with smoking.

Davison et al. say consistency theory and utility theory are not necessarily opposed to each other and can be reconciled. They say:

> One way to do this is by reference to the fact that most people seem to need reassurance that their ideas and attitudes are correct. Because they need reassurance, they seek out communications that are likely to support their existing views of the world. Thus, these supporting communications are useful. Dissonant information tends to be unsettling and unpleasant. Therefore, information of this kind may be avoided unless it has some other utility. According to this view, reassurance is only one of the needs that we commonly feel. We will pay attention to dissonant information if it helps us in some other way.[56]

Davison et al. say the uses and gratifications approach has recently become one of the most widely accepted ways of explaining why people select some content from the stream of communications and ignore other content. Uses and gratifications theory has much potential where health care communication is concerned. If it can be determined how people use the media to obtain health care information and what types of gratifications they derive from it, planning a successful health campaign might be easier. Some uses seem obvious. People want and need information about how to stay healthy. If they do suffer from a particular ailment, they are likely to seek out and absorb information about it. Quite possibly people also use media-delivered health information to confirm information they have received from physicians or friends, thus reducing uncertainty and fear. But, there could be less obvious uses and gratifications that have gone undiscovered.

AGENDA SETTING

Another hypothesis that has achieved considerable prominence since the 1960s has to do with the mass media's role in determining primarily this country's political agenda. Lowery and DeFleur say the basic idea of agenda setting can be traced to a brief passage in a book by political scientist Bernard Cohen. In 1963 he wrote: "The press may not be successful much of the time in telling people what to think, but it is stunningly successful in telling its readers what to think *about*."[57]

They say that the idea that the media provides surveillance of the environment and selectively present ideas to the public, has long been well-known. McCombs and Shaw state the agenda-setting hypothesis:

> Audiences not only learn about public issues and other matters from the media, they also learn how much importance to attach to an issue or topic from the emphasis the media place upon it.[58]

McCombs and Shaw's study of the 1968 presidential campaign found a high level of correlation between the amount of attention given to an issue in the press and the level of importance people exposed to the media assigned to the issue. The press did not persuade the people studied to adopt a particular point of view, but it did seem to make some issues more important than others—the agenda of the press became the public agenda as well.[59]

Lowery and DeFleur suggest an issue related to the agenda-setting function of the press is "the degree to which the meaning attached to issues by the public (e.g., perceived importance) play a part in formulating public policy."[60] If the press emphasizes a topic to a point where the public comes to believe that it is truly important, do political leaders then take action to "do something" about the issue? There is some recent evidence that this does happen. The news media "uncovered" the terrible drought in Africa, which was causing starvation of thousands of people. Ultimately, Congress sent aid (both money and food supplies and even military assistance). Watergate is usually the classic example given. Whether the public truly understood the realities of the case, the topic was increasingly seen as important to a point where a U.S. President left office in disgrace and under threat of impeachment.[61] Also, the level of concern the public has about the spread of

AIDS also appears to grow and wane with the amount of media space devoted to current trends in the spread of the disease and "new" treatments.

At least one study suggests that the agenda of the press can be influenced by forces outside the impact of journalistic norms, the effects of social forces within the newsroom itself, and the influence of other reporters from other newspapers. Kanervo and Kanervo offer the following summary:

> Gandy suggests that large corporations and industries exert a powerful influence on the mass media by subsidizing the cost of information-gathering through data analysis, news releases and press conferences.[62] Cutlip found 35% of newspaper content came from public relations handouts from various organizations, agencies and offices.[63] Olien, Donohue and Tichenor suggest newspaper and television coverage of an environmental issue they were studying generally occurred after interest groups defined the problem and began publicity campaigns.[64] Smith found that general public opinion on recreation and health care influenced a newspaper's agenda rather than the other way around.[65] Weaver and Elliott discovered newspaper coverage of city council meetings in a small city pretty much mirrored the agenda established by the council itself.[66]

Agenda-setting is relevant to this study because of the recent debate about health care reform. Although it could be argued that health care was a political issue that triggered media coverage, the media have long been concerned with health care topics and were touting both the strengths and weaknesses of the American health care system before Bill Clinton was elected president. Obviously, the President's concern for health care reform led to far more scrutiny by the media than would otherwise have been expected. Whether this led to increased awareness and understanding by the public is open to debate. Today, however, it is clear that health care reform is no longer on the agenda of politicians, the media or the public.

This theory implies that it also is possible for grass-roots movements to influence media coverage. Therefore, anyone who plans and implements health care promotions should know how to write press releases and court media attention.

KNOWLEDGE GAP HYPOTHESIS

Davison et al. say there are indications that the media accentuate individual differences based on education and income. Researchers have established that members of American society who are better educated take more advantage of new sources of information than those who are less educated. As a result, a "knowledge gap" develops, giving better educated and usually more affluent people even more of an advantage than they had before. Tichenor, Donohue, and Olien say:

> For example, if newspapers emphasize information on health and medicine and carry more articles on these topics, the better- educated will learn more, even though it is the less-educated who are in greater need of the information.[67]

However, there is evidence that when publicity is intense, especially when controversy is involved, the less-educated tend to catch up and narrow the gap in the information level.[68] Becker et al. found, for example, that the Ford-Carter debates in 1976 lessened the knowledge gap because the less-educated learned more about the candidates and issues than did the well-educated group.[69]

The debate among social scientists is this: Do the mass media preserve the status quo by reinforcing existing values, increasing the power of those who already have power, and focusing attention on subjects of interest to the elite, or do they promote social change through their capacity to help new interest groups and political movements to form, to acquaint people with ideas and life-styles other than their own, and to focus attention on grievances and injustices?

McQuail also points out that generally the higher the social status (often associated with education and income levels), the greater the social and economic power, the greater access to and control over the processes of communication.[70]

This theory suggests that there will be a difference in knowledge about health issues and health care among people from different education and income groups.

DIFFUSION OF INFORMATION

The next and, in some ways, the most important communication theory to be discussed is the diffusion of innovations theory, which Rogers articulated. His theory is necessary to this discussion because it explains much about the way new or "innovative" products and ideas are spread throughout mass society and because much of advertising theory and strategy has borrowed from this theory to design ads and sell products.

This study is especially interested in how information is diffused because much of health care communication is concerned with transmitting "new" treatments, technology and research findings to the public. A great deal of this information is transmitted to the public and from physician to physician through the mass media.

Rogers points out that there is much interest in the diffusion process because "getting a new idea adopted, even when it has obvious advantages, is often very difficult. There is a wide gap in many fields between what is known and what is actually put into use."[71] He offers in his book, *Diffusion of Innovations*, the following example of a diffusion campaign that failed. The public health service in Peru attempted to convince villagers to boil their drinking water. The agency wanted Nelida, a local health worker to persuade the housewives of Los Molinos to add water boiling to their pattern of daily behavior. Although Nelida spent two years visiting families, the majority (95%) never began boiling their water.[72]

Rogers concluded that the campaign failed for a number of reasons. First, local tradition linked hot foods with illness and boiling water makes it less "cold" and appropriate only for the sick. He emphasized that "an important factor affecting the adoption rate of any innovation is its compatibility with the values, beliefs, and past experiences of the social system."[73] One of the women who did adopt water boiling was somewhat of an outsider in the village and accepted the practice primarily because she wanted Nelida's approval. This underscores the importance of interpersonal networks in the adoption and rejection of an innovation, Rogers says.[74]

Nelida also worked with the wrong housewives according to Rogers. Her target women were not respected as social models while some of the women she ignored were village opinion leaders who could have activated local networks to spread the information. Nelida, herself, was viewed by poor families as a snoop and was distrusted as an outsider. She achieved her best results with middle-class women like herself. Rogers says this indicates that "how potential adopters view the change agent affects their willingness to adopt his or her ideas," and that more effective communication occurs "with those who are more similar to change agents."[75]

Rogers first offers the following definitions:

> *Diffusion* is the process by which an innovation is communicated through certain channels over time among the members of a social system.
> *Communication* is a process in which participants create and share information with one another in order to reach a mutual understanding.
> *Uncertainty* is the degree to which a number of alternatives are perceived with respect to the occurrence of an event and the relative probability of these alternatives.
> An *innovation* is an idea, practice, or object that is perceived as new by an individual or other unit of adoption. . . . If the idea seems new to the individual, it is an innovation.[76]

Rogers says that diffusion is "a kind of social change, defined as the process by which alteration occurs in the structure and function of a social system."[77] Social change occurs when new ideas are invented, diffused, and are adopted or rejected, leading to certain consequences.

According to Rogers, the uncertainty that occurs when people are trying to decide whether to adopt an innovation results in "information seeking" and "information- processing" activity in which the individual is motivated to reduce uncertainly about the advantages and disadvantages of the innovation.[78]

Obviously, in American society, some innovations are adopted rather quickly, while others may take much longer to catch on. Several communication innovations, such as VCRs, personal computers, CDs and telephone answering machines, have rather quickly found their way into American homes, while satellite dishes and cable television have been adopted in smaller numbers or have taken much longer. Cable television required physical cable to be laid before connection is possible. Dishes are both expensive and somewhat unsightly. The technological innovations that have been adopted more quickly basically require a consumer willing to pay for and learn how to use the equipment. Therefore, there are five characteristics of innovations that influence the rate at which (or even whether) an innovation is adopted:

1. *Relative advantage* is the degree to which an innovation is perceived as better than the idea it supersedes. . . . The greater the perceived relative advantage of an innovation, the more rapid its rate of adoption is going to be.

2. *Compatibility* is the degree to which an innovation is perceived as being consistent with the existing values, past experiences, and needs of potential adopters. An idea that is not compatible with the prevalent values and norms of a social system will not be adopted as rapidly as an innovation that is compatible.

3. *Complexity* is the degree to which an innovation is perceived as difficult to understand and use. . . . In general, new ideas that are simpler to understand will be adopted more rapidly than innovations that require the adopter to develop new skills and understandings.

4. *Trialability* is the degree to which an innovation may be experimented with on a limited basis. New ideas that can be tried on the installment plan will generally be adopted more quickly than innovations that are not divisible. . . .

5. *Observability* is the degree to which the results of an innovation are visible to others. The easier it is for individuals to see the results of an innovation, the more likely they are to adopt.[79]

In his discussion of communication channels, Rogers says this is the means by which messages get from one individual to another. He says the process involves:

> (1) an innovation, (2) an individual or other unit of adoption that has knowledge of, or experience with using, the innovation, (3) another individual or other unit that does not yet have knowledge of the innovation, and (4) a communication channel connecting the two units.[80]

Rogers also defined five categories that describe various groups of people involved in the adoption process. *Innovators* are active information seekers who have a high degree of mass media exposure and whose interpersonal networks extend over a wide area. They are able to cope with higher levels of uncertainty about an innovation than are other adopter categories.[81] Next in line are *early adopters* followed by *early majority, late majority,* and *laggards.*[82] When television sets first became available, for example, only the innovators purchased sets which they shared with neighbors and friends. Early adopters would be the next group to purchase sets which they also shared with friends and neighbors. Eventually, more people had sets than did not (early majority) and finally, all but a few had sets (late majority). The laggards, obviously, were the last to purchase a set or perhaps never purchased a set at all. It is expected that innovators and early adopters are likely to be those members of a society who are the most highly educated and who have the economic means to "invest" in new methods or ideas. The laggards are on the opposite end of the spectrum and are the most likely to be poorly educated and to lack economic means.

Rogers says that innovators may not be the most influential persons in the diffusion process because they may be perceived as "a deviant from the social system" resulting in "low credibility." Opinion leaders, therefore, are the most likely to influence the attitudes and/or behavior of other individuals in the social system.[83] Opinion leaders can persuade others to adopt or not adopt the innovation under scrutiny. Therefore, campaigns are most likely to succeed if opinion leaders are identified and used in the diffusion process.

Diffusion studies generally focus on the positive aspects of the process. That is, "innovations" are considered to be positive and good for the social system. Obviously, in the health area this has not always been the case. Insecticides have been promoted and then adopted to produce better crops. But the overuse of insecticides has lead to ground water pollution and absorption into the food chain. Many pesticides have now been banned because of damage to animals and humans. Also, fad diets, diet pills, steroids and other drugs have been misused by great numbers of people even though there are potentiaily serious health problems associated with them.

This theory suggests that health care promotions must keep the above five characteristics of innovations in health care in mind when formulating mass media messages.

NETWORK ANALYSIS

Rogers also has been instrumental in the formation of network analysis, a recent paradigm in communication research. Rogers and Kincaid repudiate linear models of communication in favor of the convergence model and network analysis. "Convergence," they point out, "is the tendency for two or more individuals to move toward one point, or for one individual to move toward another, and to unite in a common interest or focus."[84]

Kincaid defines communication as "a process of convergence in which information is shared by participants in order to reach a mutual understanding."[85] The authors further say a personal network is "composed of other individuals with whom one interacts, whether they belong to identifiable 'groups' or not." Because no two individuals have the same interpersonal communication pattern, codes and concepts among individuals may be similar but never identical.[86] At the core of this paradigm is information, which Rogers and Kincaid define as "a difference in matter-energy which affects uncertainty in a situation where a choice exists among a set of alternatives." They point out:

> At the psychological level, a choice is made by the application of concepts. The greater the number and variety of concepts available in an individual's cognitive system, the greater the individual's ability to perceive differences in the environment.[87]

The authors say that "shared" information can lead to mutual understanding, mutual agreement, and collective action. Thus, they say:

> Information and mutual understanding are the dominant components of our convergence model of communication. Information-processing at the individual level involves perceiving, interpreting, understanding, believing, and action, which creates—potentially, at least—new information for further processing. When information is *shared* by two or more participants, information-processing may lead to mutual understanding, mutual agreement, and collective action.[88]

Their convergence model consists of three levels of reality or abstraction: 1) the physical level, 2) the psychological level, and 3) the social level. They state that "the primary purpose of human communication is to define and to understand reality so that other human purposes can be achieved."[89]

Rogers and Kincaid contend that the most important characteristic of the information-sharing process is the communication circuit, or network of circuits, which connect people within a system. They describe this circuit as a "circular loop, with the capacity for a continuous two-way exchange of information." This loop is necessary for feedback, which the authors believe is essential for communication and which they describe as "a process over time":

> When several cycles of information-exchange are considered, and the information is observed as changing over time, then feedback must be conceptualized as a process, and not as knowledge held at one point in time. To avoid the confusion that currently exists regarding this distinction, we must use the concepts of convergence and divergence.[90]

The authors say that the convergence model and network analysis fit so well together because in network analysis, no sharp distinction is made between source and receiver. Rather communication flows among "transceivers" in the network, each of whom are both, in turn, transmitters and receivers. Therefore, they recommend one or more of the following research procedures:

1. Identify *cliques* (subsystem whose elements interact with each other relatively more frequently than with other members of the communication system) within the total system and determine how these subgroupings affect communication behavior in the system.
2. Identify *certain specialized communication roles* such as liaisons (individual who links two or more cliques in a system, but who is not a member of any clique), bridges (an individual who links two or more cliques in a system from his or her position as a member of one of the cliques), and isolates.
3. Measure various *communication structural indexes* (like communication connectedness, for example) for individuals, dyads, personal networks, cliques, or entire systems.
4. Measure *communications links* through survey sociometry, observation, and unobtrusive methods.[91]

Brenner suggests that Q methodology also fits well with the convergence model and diffusion research. He discusses why medical information systems (MIS), computer-based systems for integrating patient records, laboratory test results, and patient management data, were not being diffused successfully. A classical diffusion analysis focused on the characteristics of the innovation failed to explain the failure, Brenner says. Q methodology was used to determine physicians' relevant concourses, a term Stephenson used to describe the way individuals associate information and attitudes. The Q study yielded three factors, or physicians' concourses. The conclusion was that physicians were concerned about surrendering part of the control of their patients, about the system intruding between them and their patients, and about changing their roles in what they regarded as inappropriate ways.[92] Brenner points out:

> ... the application of Q permitted the analysis of the important structures of the adoption situation, a situation that other researchers despaired at attempting to analyze because the relationships are ever-changing. . . .[93]

Further, Brenner says all of the concepts that Rogers and Kincaid identify as measuring communication structure at the individual, clique, and system level are explicated in the Q factors:

1. *Connectedness*: The degree to which a unit is linked to other units.
2. *Integration*: the degree to which the units linked to the focal unit are linked to each other.
3. *Diversity*: The degree to which the units linked to the focal unit are heterogeneous in some variable.
4. *Openness*: The degree to which a unit exchanges information with its environment. [94]

Brenner advocates the use of Q methodology in diffusion research and network analysis as part of the paradigms and research methods that Rogers and Kincaid describe.

This model, then, integrates many facets of other models. There is a concern with physical proximity in terms of setting up communication networks, with opinion leaders, with audience reaction (divergence or convergence), and with feedback and communication loops. Health care campaign planners should be concerned with these elements as well.

CONCLUSIONS

The most striking change in communication theory during the twentieth century has been the perception of the audience as active rather than passive.

This, of course, means that the view of the mass media has changed from all powerful to influential to varying degrees. Do the media have an effect on the audience in general? Of course, they do in the sense that information can be presented quickly and public opinion can be molded to some extent. The difficulty is that the boundaries of influence are not well defined and perhaps never will be. Nearly everyone in America can learn virtually overnight about scandals and heinous crimes, but there appears to be little evidence that the judicial system is swayed. The health care system has been warning for years that smoking is dangerous to a person's health, yet thousands of people begin smoking every year. Also, the media do not exist in a vacuum. Government and business offer controls in the form of press releases and access to information. Relatives, friends, neighbors, and coworkers put pressure on members of their spheres to believe certain things and behave in certain ways. Individuals filter and sort information either seeking or avoiding information that interests them, serves them or pleasures them in some manner.

The ultimate conclusion is that planners of media campaigns, in particular health campaigns, must examine many approaches and variables, study the target audience and choose approaches that offer the most promise for catching the audience's attention, leaving a lasting impression, provide needed information in an absorbable form and provide a model of action in the hopes that the behavior of *some* who are exposed to it will change in the desired direction. The next chapter will look more thoroughly at the process of planning a media campaign based on what is known about the health needs of African Americans and communication theory.

NOTES

1. Melvin L. DeFleur and Sandra Ball-Rokeach, *Theories of Mass Communication*, 5th ed., (White Plains, NY: Longman Inc., 1989), 181.

2. Ibid., 186.

3. Ibid., 117.

4. Shearon Lowery and Melvin L. DeFleur, *Milestones in Mass Communication Research: Media Effects* (White Plains, NY: Longman Inc., 1983), 24.

5. Ibid., 24-25.

6. DeFleur and Ball-Rokeach, 180.

7. Ibid.

8. W. Phillips Davison, James Boylan, and Frederick T.C. Yu, *Mass Media Systems & Effects,* 2d Ed., (New York: CBS College Publishing, 1982), 187.

9. Ibid., 189.

10. Ibid., 190.

11. Ibid., 211.

12. Ibid.

13. Melvin L. DeFleur, *Theories of Mass Communication* (New York: David McKay Company, Inc., 1966), 121.

14. Davison et al., 169.

15. Ibid.

16. DeFleur and Ball-Rokeach, 196.

17. DeFleur, 121.

18. DeFleur and Ball-Rokeach, 197.

19. Ibid.

20. Davison et al., 186.

21. Ibid., 187.

22. Lowery and DeFleur, 26.

23. Ibid.

24. DeFleur and Ball-Rokeach, 181.

25. Judith Sylvester, "Media Research Bureau Black Newspaper Readership Report," Sears Foundation/National Newspaper Publishers Association report, (University of Missouri: June 24, 1993).

26. Lowery and DeFleur, 152.

27. Ibid., 154.

28. Ibid.

29. Ibid., 165.

30. Ibid.

31. Ibid.

32. Ibid., 166.

33. Ibid.

34. Ibid.

35. Ibid., 27.

36. Ibid., 27-28.

37. Ibid., 28-29.

38. Davison et al., 150.

39. Ibid.

40. Ibid.

41. Ibid.

42. Ibid., 156.

43. DeFleur and Ball-Rokeach, 311.

44. Ibid., 311-312.

45. Ibid., 313.

46. Ibid., 314.

47. Ibid.

48. Ibid.

49. Lowery and DeFleur, 373.

50. Ibid.

51. Davison et al., 159.

52. William Stephenson, *The Play Theory of Mass Communication* (Chicago: University of Chicago Press, 1967), 48.

53. Ibid., 374.

54. Davison et al., 159.

55. Elihu Katz, Michael Gurevitch, and Hadassah Haas, "On the Uses of the Mass Media for Important Things," *American Sociological Review* 38, (1973): 164-181.

56. Davison et al., 159.

57. Bernard Cohen, *The Press and Foreign Policy* (Princeton, NJ: Princeton University Press, 1963), 13.

58. Maxwell E. McCombs and Donald L. Shaw, "Structuring the 'Unseen Environment,'" *Journal of Communication* 26(2), (Spring, 1976): 18.

59. DeFleur and Ball-Rokeach, 264.

60. Lowery and DeFleur, 381.

61. Ibid.

62. Oscar Gandy, *Beyond Agenda Setting: Information Subsidies and Public Policies* (Norwood, N.J.: Ablex Publishing Company, 1982) cited in Ellen Williamson Kanervo and David W. Kanervo, *Journalism Quarterly*, 66(2), 308-309.

63. Scott M. Cutlip, "Third of Newspapers' Content PR Inspired," *Editor & Publisher*, (May 26, 1962)cited in Ellen Williamson Kanervo and David W. Kanervo, *Journalism Quarterly*, 66(2), 309.

64. Clarice N. Olien, George A. Donohue, and Phillip Tichenor, "Media and Stages of Social Conflict," *Journalism Monographs* 90, (November 1984) cited in Kanervo and Kanervo, 309.

65. Kim Smith, "Newspaper Coverage and Public Concern about Community Issues: A Time-Series Analysis," *Journalism Monographs* 101 (February 1987) cited in Ellen Williamson Kanervo and David W. Kanervo, *Journalism Quarterly* 66(2), 309.

66. David Weaver and Swanzy Nimley Elliott, "Who Sets the Agenda for the Media? A Study of Local Agenda Building," *Journalism Quarterly* 62 (Spring 1985) cited in Ellen Williamson Kanervo and David W. Kanervo, *Journalism Quarterly* 66(2), 309.

67. Phillip J. Tichenor, G.A. Donohue, and C.N. Olien, "Mass Media Flow and the Differential Growth of Knowledge," *Public Opinion Quarterly,* 34, (1970): 159-170 quoted in Davison et al., 211.

68. Phillip J. Tichenor et al., *Community Conflict and the Press*, (Beverly Hills, Ca.: Sage, 1980), 49.

69. Lee B. Becker, et al., "Debates' Effects on Voters' Understanding of Candidates and Issues," *The Presidential Debates: Media, Electoral, and Policy Perspectives,* eds. George F. Bishop, Robert G. Meadow, and Marilyn Jackson-Beeck, (New York: Praeger, 1978), 138.

70. Davison, 196.

71. Everett M. Rogers, *Diffusion of Innovations*, 3d ed., (New York: The Free Press, Div. Macmillan Publishing Co., Inc., 1983), 1.

72. Ibid., 4.

73. Ibid.

74. Ibid.

75. Ibid., 4-5.

76. Ibid., 5, 6, 11.

77. Ibid., 6.

78. Ibid., 13.

79. Ibid., 15-16.

80. Ibid., 17.

81. Ibid., 22.

82. Ibid.

83. Ibid., 27.

84. Everett M. Rogers and D. Lawrence Kincaid, *Communication Networks: Toward a New Paradigm for Research* (New York: The Free Press, 1981), 62.

85. Ibid., 35.

86. Ibid., 44-45.

87. Ibid., 54.

88. Ibid., 56.

89. Ibid., 54, 63.

90. Ibid., 61-62.

91. Ibid., 38, 97.

92. Donald J. Brenner, "Beyond Diffusion: Network Analysis and Q," Paper presented at the second annual Conference on the Scientific Study of Subjectivity, Columbia, Mo., July, 1986., 6-7.

93. Ibid., 7.

94. Ibid.

CHAPTER IV

Health Campaigns:
A Marketing Perspective

In the forward to his 1967 report on medical communication, William Stephenson says:

> There is no lack of the means of communication—of books, brochures, pamphlets, films, telephones, lecturers, close-circuit television and the rest. There is no lack of faith, also, in the belief that "to communicate is the beginning of understanding." This report, however, suggests the opposite, that "to understand is the beginning of communication."[1]

This chapter is concerned both with understanding and communicating in the form of a health care campaign. It is important to note that although much has been written about the successes and failures of health campaigns, few of the books and articles reviewed specifically deal with the problems of designing campaigns that target minorities. Apparently, there have been few attempts to examine the approaches necessary to accomplish such a task. Therefore, general principles will be outlined here, and specific recommendations for designing a health campaign that targets African Americans will be detailed in following chapters.

CAMPAIGN DEFINITIONS AND ELEMENTS

Wright and Warner's define a campaign in the following manner:

> The word "campaign" is derived from the medieval Latin word *compania*, or level country and was used to describe battle maneuvers executed on the

Plains. Though the principles of attaining specific objectives in advertising campaigns, political campaigns, or civil rights campaigns are basically the same, historically greater study has been given them as military campaign principles.[2]

Kirkpatrick defines a campaign as "an organized series of advertising messages . . . an orderly, planned effort consisting of related but self-contained and independent advertisements."[3] Further, he says a campaign has a single theme or keynote idea, a single objective or goal, and a group of individual advertisements that purposely resemble each other.

Flay and Burton define a communication campaign as "an integrated series of communication activities, using multiple operations and channels, aimed at populations or large target audiences, usually of long duration, with a clear purpose."[4]

Backer and Rogers say their concept of a health communication campaign follows from the basic definition offered by Rogers and Storey in 1988:

1.   A campaign is purposive and seeks to influence individuals.
2.   A campaign is aimed at a large audience.
3.   A campaign has a more or less specifically defined time limit.
4.   A campaign involves an organized set of communication activities.[5]

Devine and Hirt define an information campaign as "organized attempts to influence another's beliefs about, attitudes toward, and/or behaviors with respect to some object (e.g., product, issue, persons, etc.) through the use of mass media or other communication channels." They suggest that their definition implies campaign effectiveness can be assessed against a variety of criteria.[6]

Flay and Burton emphasize that although there are many similarities, campaigns promoting products differ from health campaigns on several dimensions (adapted from McCron & Budd, 1981):

> *Type of change expected.* Many health campaigns aim to change fundamental behaviors, whereas most product advertising aims to mobilize an existing prodispostion, as in switching brands.

Amount of change expected. Health campaigns aim to change a large proportion of the population, and often in large ways. Product advertising campaigners are usually satisfied with small shifts in market share.

Time frame of promised benefits. Health campaigns usually ask their target audience to wait for delayed statistical probabilities, such as reduced likelihood of eventual illness or a few additional years of life. Product advertisers promise immediate certainty and satisfaction.

Presentation of the product. Advertisers can dress up their product in an exaggerated fashion, for a certain amount of deception (e.g., imagery advertising associating social success with buying a particular brand of Scotch) seems to be acceptable to audiences. On the other hand, health campaigners avoid overselling the benefits of a behavior or treatment and the ease of their acquisition.

Available budgets. Commercial advertisers often have massive budgets, while health campaigners usually operate on relatively minuscule monetary resources.

Trustworthiness. People often distrust commercial advertising, even though they may be affected by it. Health campaigns cannot allow distrust to develop, although there appears to be some skepticism of government-sponsored health messages.

Level of evaluation. Advertisers stress formative market research conducted before a campaign. Many health campaigns still ignore evaluation; when research is performed, it tends to be summative evaluation carried out after the campaign.[7]

Flay and Burton also outline seven steps necessary for an effective campaign:

1. Develop and use high quality messages, sources, and channels.
2. Disseminate to the target audience.
3. Gain and keep the attention of the audience.
4. Encourage favorable interpersonal communication about the issue.
5. Cause changes in behaviors of individuals, along with awareness, knowledge, opinions, attitudes, feelings, normative beliefs, intentions, or skills.
6. Cause broader societal changes.
7. Obtain knowledge of effects through summative evaluation.[8]

Mass media approaches, community-based activities, and individual interactions are important aspects of a campaign, as Backer and Rogers say:

Modern health communication campaigns use a variety of approaches to deliver health messages to their targeted audiences. . . . The mass media component of health communication campaigns typically is an important one, and approaches ranging from network television public-service announcements, to public affairs "specials" on cable television, to print ads in newspapers, and many others are all part of the modern campaign designer's "tool kit."

. . . (M)ost campaigns use multiple media, in conjunction with community-based and interpersonal methods of message delivery and promotion of knowledge, attitude, or behavior change. Some, such as former First Lady Nancy Reagan's "Just Say No" drug abuse prevention campaign for children in the 1980s, become so visible that they become part of the popular culture. Others, such as the Stanford Heart Disease Prevention Program, have a much lower public profile nationally, although they may be highly visible in their local area.[9]

Olins, one of Stephenson's students, has examined the concepts involved in an advertising campaign. He points out that a campaign is a part of a wider set of marketing activities that include production, distribution, servicing, and especially facilitation.[10] He says that because advertising is a form of communication, the degree of acceptance of the message depends upon the level to which the individual targeted will be able to identify with it. Otherwise, the individual will become either critical of the message or ambivalent toward it.

Cox, in the *Harvard Business Review*,[11] provides the following three assumptions:

1. Ads mainly reinforce pre-disposition; consumers are therefore pre-selective vis-a-vis ads.
2. We cannot assume that all consumers are different in predispositions, or all alike. There cannot be one ad campaign, therefore, applicable to everyone. Instead, there are "groups," "segments," or "special interest" components—we talk therefore of the teen market, of brand loyalties, etc.
3. Changing these "groups" is beyond the scope of ad campaigns, though minor opinions can be altered, and consumers without brand loyalty may switch as the result of advertising.

Olins indicates that Stephenson's theory of communication sees advertising from a subjective rather than an objective viewpoint. "The concern is with what people say, what images, wishes, and fantasies they have about consuming, buying and advertisements—as well as about such facts as matters to this communication," he says.[12]

Wiebe says basic communication principles include:

1. Consumers are apperceptive, taking notice only of what is of interest to them; they identify with what interests them.
2. Interests are schematical and many consumers have much the same schemata: i.e., we can identify "groups" of consumers with much the same interests.
3. Ad messages have to be such as "groups" can identify with.
4. If "groups" can identify positively with an ad message (or the product or service) the result is *communication-pleasure*.
5. If "groups" cannot identify with an ad message the result is *communication-pain* (displeasure often resulting in distortion of the message, because of conditions of self-worth).
6. Messages themselves do not lead to action (i.e., buying), but only to communication: buying and consuming is effected by facilitating mechanisms.[13]

Salmon emphasizes that whether cause of death or illness is selected to become the focus of a health campaign may rest on a number of political as well as medical factors. He says:

> Given that no single definition of a problem is uniquely accurate, the power to control the framing or defining of an issue is of paramount importance if an organization is to gain acceptance of its proposed solution. Without question, this power resides disproportionately with government, corporations and other institutions possessing legitimacy, social power and resources and access to the mass media. Yet campaigns, in and of themselves are not inherently weapons of the social elite; some campaigns are conducted by socially disadvantaged groups seeking to induce extensive systemic change.[14]

Salmon points out that other campaigns are sponsored by organizations "seeking to alter basic societal assumptions, laws and norms, and seeking to locate the origin of social problems within the system."[15]

Obviously, from the definitions presented, it is clear that a campaign with the goal of improving the health of African Americans (the target group) should involve a clear set of goals and objectives that would include changes in knowledge, attitudes, and behaviors during a specified time period. Such a campaign should use both the mass media and community organizations for maximum results. The mass media component should include advertising techniques to help design and "sell" messages. Political and social agendas also should be considered whenever possible.

REASONS HEALTH CAMPAIGNS FAIL

Lack of attention to any of the campaign components mentioned above can result in an ineffective effort. Wallack, for example, offers a major discourse on the difficulties of creating successful health care campaigns. He focuses his attention on campaigns concerning drinking, smoking, and drugs because of their common characteristics:

> First, they address major social or health problems (or sometimes, like the anti-marijuana campaigns of the 1930s, the problem may be primarily political) and often these problems have special qualities of intractability. Second, virtually all of these campaigns have been oriented toward the general population and traditionally have utilized all available channels of mass media. Third, implicitly or explicitly, it is expected that these programs will cause a detectable (measurable) level of behavior change in a detectable part of the population. Fourth, all campaigns are subject to some level of evaluation, whether it be formal or informal. Fifth, perhaps except for planned campaigns to reduce illicit drug use these campaigns usually take place in a relatively hostile environment of strong vested interests.[16]

He says that for 20 years programs apparently assumed that reaching the general population solely by means of mass media was sufficient, as opposed to previous campaigns that utilized mass media plus grass-roots participation techniques. "A specific focus in behavior, however, is seldom seen and most often campaigns seek to increase knowledge or change attitudes, assuming that behavior change will follow," he says.[17] Wallack says in health campaigns various types of behavior change are advocated. Campaigns can ask for adoption of new behaviors. They can serve only to remind, reinforce, or slightly modify existing behavior. Others do not expect people to necessarily give up a valued behavior altogether but might ask them to adopt a functionally equivalent or alternative behavior or they might advocate risk minimization.[18]

Wallack also notes there are several ways to evaluate a campaign. These can range from rather low-level efforts that can be subjective statements by program participants, administrators or sponsors to high level efforts that use experimental designs and scientific rigor. The latter may include exposure or recall studies, and surveys that seek to measure knowledge, opinion and attitude change, and/or behavior changes.

Wallack says that campaigns do not take place in a vacuum "but confront strongly vested financial interests and deep-rooted well-established values." He says that problems such as smoking, drinking, and drug-taking behaviors have two important characteristics:

> First, they occur to a relative minority of our population (even though that minority might number millions of people). Second, they result in significant part from arrangements that are providing substantial benefits or advantages to a majority or powerful minority of citizens. Thus solving or minimizing these problems requires painful losses, the restructuring of society and the acceptance of new burdens is the most powerful and the numerous on behalf of the least powerful or least numerous.[19]

Wallack says mass media programs that change individual-level behavior have two major components: a theory or theoretical model of how to attain the goal (behavior change) and a method for implementing a program. If the campaign fails to achieve its goals, then either or both of the components could be faulty. As Wallack says:

> Thus a program failure may be due to either faulty implementation or an invalid model of behavior change, or both. If we assume that both of these key assumptions have to be valid then we can see all other things being equal, that the odds against success are stacked. Given the methodological problems to which virtually all field evaluations are prone, the odds against finding success, if it does occur, reduce further the probability of a successful program.[20]

Wallack also implies that programs will be most successful if mass media messages or advertising show how the behavior being advocated or the service being offered will somehow satisfy a pre-existing need or desire of the audience member. For example, if someone has already decided to lose weight, an advertisement for a hospital weight loss program will probably appeal more to that person than to someone who is at or below his or her ideal weight. Likewise, a weight-loss program, no matter how well advertised and promoted, will not succeed if there is no market for it in the first place. Also, attempting to change ingrained habits, such as ethnic diets and cigarette smoking habits, can be very difficult, especially in a short amount of time. As Wallack says, "Evidence seems to bear out the related concept that advertising is more effective in gaining new users within an existing market (market share) than in recruiting users not currently in the market (market growth)."[21]

Wallack also advocates the need for supplementation, usually in the form of interpersonal contact, to augment the use of mass media. He cites the Stanford Heart Study[22] as an example of supplementation. Although mass media alone showed some positive effects, the mass media plus personalized instruction enhanced considerably the effectiveness of the mass media in reducing the risk of heart disease.

Another difficulty with measuring likely attitude and behavior change is that there can be major differences between what people say and what people do. An example is LaPiere's classic 1934 study of prejudice that reported on his cross-country travels with a young Chinese couple during the 1930-1932 period. Out of 251 transactions for accommodations and other services the travelers were only refused service once although responses to a questionnaire sent to the establishments six months later more than 90% indicated they would not accept members of the Chinese race as guests.[23] Deutscher's critical review finds "no reason to expect to find congruence between attitudes and action and every reason to expect to find discrepancies between them."[24]

Wicker reviewed the relationship of verbal and overt behavioral responses to attitudes and concludes:

> Taken as a whole these studies suggest that it is considerably more likely that attitudes will be unrelated or only slightly related to overt behaviors than that attitudes will be closely related to actions.[25]

However, Wallack says those who dispute the lack of attitude-behavior consistency either view attitude-behavior relationships as multivariate rather than bivariate or believe that the concept of attitudes is ill-defined resulting in measurement problems. It is also possible that attitude concepts are poorly understood and incorrectly measured.[26]

After a review of the attitude-behavior literature, Ajzen and Fishbein[27] developed a theory that suggests attitude and behavioral entities consist of four elements: the action, the target at which the action is directed, the context in which the action is performed, and the time at which it is performed. Their conclusion is that if the attitudinal and behavioral entities are identical in their elements, there is correspondence. However, attitudes are measured with reference to target or target combined with action but not to action, context and time. This may be one reason for low attitude-behavior correlations.[28] Their review of the research concludes that there is a direct positive relationship between degree of correspondence and attitude-behavior relations and contrary to past research suggesting inconsistency between attitudes and behavior:

> The findings concerning the relation between attitude and behavior only appear to be inconsistent. A person's attitude has a consistently strong relation with his or her behavior when it is directed at the same target and when it involves the same action.[29]

They found that attitude-behavior relations increase in strength when appropriate measures are used.[30]

Wallack says the lack of evidence to support attitude change/behavior change consistency is problematic for public information programs because "it is difficult to justify the use of attitude change as an operational definition of behavior change as many public information and education programs have done."[31]

To be sure that campaign evaluations are measuring the correct dimensions, planners should specify what they want people to know, what they want people to believe, what they want people to do as a result of the campaign and what they want to know themselves as the result of the evaluation. Finally, Wallack says the focus of evaluation should include avenues of inquiry beyond just individual level behavior change.[32]

SOCIAL MARKETING

An approach to designing and implementing information campaigns that attempts to answer Wallack's criticisms is social marketing. This approach will guide most of the discussion that follows in this chapter. Manoff states that the power of social marketing is its use of a public voice—the mass media, the most potent of all.[33]

Salmon traces the beginning of social marketing to 1952 when G.D. Wiebe's asked, "Why can't you sell brotherhood and rational thinking like you sell soap?"[34] Manoff adds several other steps in the development process.[35] First is the 1969 White House Conference on Food, Nutrition, and Health that included a panel on "Popular Education: How to Reach Disadvantaged Groups Through the Media of Mass Communications. This conference tentatively acknowledged marketing's possibilities in health promotion. Next, Manoff says several efforts in developing countries won the support of USAID, the Ford Foundation, and CARE to carry out mass media campaigns employing advertising techniques, message design and testing, media analysis, effectiveness tracking, etc. Then, during the United Nations conference at Alma-Ata in 1978 the principles of primary health care were officially enunciated. Manoff says:

> Alma-Ata also underscored the role of the community in programs for its benefit and repudiated the doctrine of health paternalism implicit in plans designed unilaterally by authorities and handed down to communities as fais accomplis. These principles of program integration and community-based planning would revise for all time the strategies of public health promotion. Though few realized it at the time, these changes were soon to win for marketing an acceptance undreamed of a few short years before.[36]

Salmon identifies three phases of the social marketing process:

1. The definition of a social condition as a social problem meriting intervention.
2. Implementation of campaign activities.
3. Evaluation of the effectiveness of those activities.

Atkin and Wallack say "social marketing has evolved as a popular approach that attempts to apply advertising and marketing principles to the 'selling' of positive health behaviors."[37] They say:

> In general, social marketing provides a framework in which marketing concepts are integrated with social-influence theories to develop programs better able to accomplish behavior change goals. It borrows the planning variables from marketing—product, price, promotion, place—and reinterprets these for a particular health issue.[38]

Communication and social-psychological theories are used to develop the social marketing program, and marketing techniques are used to develop messages and implement the program. Usually, social marketing also includes local organizations and interpersonal networks to influence behavior change. As Atkin and Wallack point out, "a key principle of social marketing is the reduction of psychological, social, economic, and practical distance between the consumer and the behavior."[39]

Similar to other campaign techniques, social marketing involves a definition of the problem and a set of objectives that can be clearly specified and implemented. The main difference between social marketing and other approaches is the emphasis on consumer needs.[40]

As Salmon indicates, "an information campaign . . . is a form of social intervention prompted by a determination that some situation represents a social problem meriting social action." Further, he says:

> Depending upon the context, this social situation can take the form of some individual or group, a change agent or agency, making such determination as: some consumers are unaware (but should not be) of some organization's service which may improve their lives; some social systems are insufficiently "advanced" or "modernized" (and should change); some individuals are engaging in behaviors which bring them pleasure, but which also have a level of risk associated with them that a change agency considers too high (so they should cease these behaviors); or some government is being unresponsive to the needs of certain groups by failing to distribute resources in a manner which a change agency considers equitable (so the government should alter its philosophy of allocation).[41]

Manoff emphasizes that there are a number of "gaps" that social marketing can bridge. The first of these is a comprehension gap that can be created by "outmoded message- design concepts" that are "cumbersome, complicated, and confusing in their focus on a device rather than on substance."[42] Confusing about food groups is the example he uses to illustrate this gap. Through the years different government agencies have advocated dividing food into first five, then seven, then four groups. Now, a new pyramid grouping is being used. Such inconsistency can confuse consumers. "Knowledge of the foods and why they are important is lost in the clutter," Manoff says.[43]

The second problem is an "awareness gap" caused by "deficiencies in message, materials, and media."[44] For example, the U.S. food stamp program in its early years was used by only 16 percent of those eligible. Manoff says that "a proper effort would have identified the barriers and set out to level them by taking the issue to the public—to rescue it from the doldrums, to keep public officials faithful, and to arouse popular awareness."[45]

The materials gap is the third problem. Manoff views this as a lack of understanding of technology, particularly the use of the media and their materials.[46]

Manoff also sees gaps between:

1. The two cultures of the target audience and the health professional.
2. Educational assumption and popular perception.
3. Educational content and such realities of the environment as deleterious practices in the marketplace.
4. The dissonant messages from responsible authorities.
5. The health care system and large numbers of the needy who are unmotivated to avail themselves of its facilities.
6. The emphasis on and competition between curative services and the rising need for prevention.[47]

Hornik is concerned with the gap between knowledge and behavior. He says:

> In the United States, the archetypal example of the knowledge-behavior gap is smoking. Smokers know they shouldn't smoke, but they do it anyway. How is the gap explained? Where there is a common reference to

physical addiction, there is much emphasis on psychological needs, including describing smoking as habitual behavior responding to environmental cues. Some note the strong association of social class with smoking and suggest that social reference groups may play some role. However, many of the essential intervention strategies, such as behavior-modification or smoking-education programs, reflect an assumption that the decision to give up smoking must be made by an individual and, implicitly, that the decision is substantially within the control of the smoker.[48]

Hornik offers five classes of "susceptibility" hypotheses to project when the knowledge-behavior link be tight and when will it be loose. First is the "structural characteristics of communities." For example, communities that are advantaged in development may provide more opportunity and knowledge which can be turned into behavior.[49]

Second is the "structural characteristics of individuals," which implies that some people are not able to turn knowledge into behavior because they lack the personal resources to undertake the practice.[50]

Third is "community social influences." Hornik says a social view of the process of behavior change implies that behavior doesn't belong only to individuals but also belongs to social groupings. He says smoking, which is substantially a social behavior, is an example.[51]

's fourth class is the "learned characteristics of individuals," which he says includes "factors such as prior knowledge and learned skills, which may be relatively open to shorter-term changes ." Finally, pinpoints the "enduring characteristics of individuals" as the fifth class. He believes it is possible that personality may make some people more innovative than others. [52]

In summary, he says that these hypotheses suggest that experience and personality "affect the ease with which one handles the concepts transmitted in a public information campaign. If one is more comfortable with the concepts, if one can fit them into preexisting cognitive schema, one can act on them more readily."[53]

Beyond the concern with gaps, there are other distinctions between marketing and social marketing. Manoff says:

Marketing is a neutral methodology and social marketing is its adaption to public imperatives. The distinction between the two is in substance and objective but not in methodology. Social marketing of public health is not to be confused with the marketing activity of the new commercial health care and hospital corporations. These are business organizations whose raison d'etre is to market health products and services for the profit of stockholders.[54]

Manoff lists the following principles for the interdisciplinary approach of social marketing:

1. Identify the health problems and the marketing and message actions required for their solution.
2. Establish priorities, select affordable efforts, and set up a deferred schedule for all others.
3. Analyze the distinct marketing/message activities needed for each problem/solution.
4. Pinpoint the target audience for each marketing/message action.
5. Conduct the necessary research on each marketing/message concept to determine current target audience attitudes and uncover potential resistance points.
6. Establish objectives for each target group and each marketing/message action.
7. Design the marketing/message actions.
8. Test the marketing/message actions for acceptability, implementation, comprehension, believability, motivation, and conviction.
9. Revise and retest the marketing/distribution and message/media patterns to achieve maximum target audience reach and message frequency.
10. Coordinate and harmonize with all ongoing related programs.
11. Track the impact of each marketing/message action and modify according to findings.[55]

Further, Manoff offers an outline of a social marketing campaign that involves strategy development, strategy formulation, strategy implementation, programming inauguration, and strategy assessment. He says the necessary resources to conduct a social marketing campaign include a research facility, the mass media, media professionals capable of analyzing and planning their use, marketing experts, creative people for message design, and materials production specialists.[56]

He also stresses the necessity of consensus building among collaborators (who often are researchers, planners, media experts, government agency representatives, and community representatives) to assist with problem definition, goal setting, and minimization of message dissonance.[57]

According to Flay and Burton, formative research, especially focus groups, is the primary tool for tailoring public communication efforts to specific audiences. Other kinds of formative research can include "analysis of the audience, so the population can be segmented into homogeneous groups; measurement of media habits of the target population, so the messages can be placed in the proper media at the proper time; and assessment of pre-existing knowledge and attitudes in the target population."[58]

Hertog et al. suggest that public health campaign planners increasingly are relying on formative analysis methods to improve the chances that community populations will adopt recommended health behavior changes.[59] They consider formative methods to include both qualitative and quantitative research methods that differentiate potential target audiences, assess the audiences' health-related needs, construct informative and persuasive messages, synthesize and integrate multiple educational strategies to effective programs, and deliver programs and messages through combinations of channels likely to be used by different audience groups.

The authors say the focus of most health interventions has either been to "educate" or to try to change behaviors. "Health professionals have been frustrated time and again by the apparent unwillingness of people to do what is good for them. This has led to a tendency to blame people for their own sickness on the one hand, and to call for government intervention on the other (for example, taxing cigarettes and making their advertisement illegal)," they say.[60] A possible reason for this is a lack of understanding of the life situations of groups in the population and their psychological, social and structural reasons for unhealthy behavior. The authors suggest members of the audience are asked to change ingrained behaviors but are not given sufficient help in making those changes. Some health campaigns seem to center on the idea, "Do this because it is good for you," which the authors say assumes that 1) behavior change is relatively easy, 2) the benefits of the change outweigh the costs, including gratification the audience receives from engaging in unhealthy behavior, and 3) the message is automatically accepted because of the assumed authority of the source. They think all these assumptions are questionable.[61]

Secondly, campaign ineffectiveness can be the result of problems with the channels used to convey the message. Hertog et al. say the intended audience may not attend to the channels or channels used to distribute the message; or the message may be drowned out by other messages in the system, including health claims from other sources, some not reliable. They suggest formative research can help deal with any or all of these concerns:

> By developing a greater understanding of the beliefs, attitudes, and behaviors of potential changers, along with an increased knowledge of the barriers to change (both personal and social), health intervention programs can be developed which will be more successful.[62]

Social marketing argues that "a focus upon the beliefs, needs, and wants of the audience, rather than that of the advocate, will lead to greater success in promoting change."[63] When using the "marketing concept," wants and needs of the consumer are identified and satisfied. Services are promoted in ways which the consumer finds relevant and useful. Hertog et al. say health marketers should focus on consumers, researching their health needs and wants, and then develop programs that meet those needs, rather than carrying on medical research and then trying to get the consumer to accept and act on the findings.[64] Social marketing recognizes that populations are not homogeneous but may be differentiated by their sociodemographic and psychological characteristics, by their needs, desires, and lifestyles, and by their motivations to act.[65] Consequently, informative and persuasive communication strategies should be developed and tailored for each subgroup in order to enhance the potential for widespread adoption of ideas or behaviors.[66]

Brown says the idea of combining interpersonal and mass media communication campaigns is not new, but perhaps underutilized. He points out that several health researchers argue that health communication is most effective when both interpersonal and mass communication campaigns are employed jointly.[67] Because mass media and interpersonal influences are interactive, they should be studied together.[68] He also suggests that health information received through media sources is often disseminated through interpersonal communication networks.[69]

In spite of its obvious advantages, Flay and Burton point out that social marketing has a number of limitations that inhibit its usefulness. They say it has been criticized as being "manipulative and theoretical suspect" because of its close relationship to more general advertising and marketing practices. Social marketing has also been criticized for promoting "single solutions to complex health problems and ignoring the conditions that give rise to and sustain disease." Flay and Burton use the example of campaigns that focus on changing individual health habits in developing countries rather than insuring a clean water supply.[70]

Furthermore, Flay and Burton say:

> Social marketing also faces the difficult task of motivating the voluntary exchange process with the consumer that is so crucial to its effectiveness. The limited success of typical health promotion programs which offer increased health status, positive image, and presume peer approval in exchange for delayed gratifications (e.g., exercise), risk of social rejection (e.g., abstinence form drugs), or physical discomfort (e.g., withdrawal from cigarettes), does not provide much basis for optimism.[71]

The sections that follow will examine various elements that can be included in a social marketing plan and relate them to possible uses in a campaign that targets African Americans.

ADVERTISING CAMPAIGN THEORY

Advertising campaign theory, obviously useful to social marketing, can be used to make health campaigns more effective. Quera, for example, says the activity of advertising boils down to "efforts to persuade people to act in certain ways." In order to make advertising work, he says "mental intercourse" is required between the originator and sender of a message and a receiver.[72] He considers the originator to be the advertiser and the receiver the potential buyer, but this concept applies equally well to the campaign planner, who in this case is interested in a service (health care) and the target audience who would be consumers of health information and services. Quera says that unless some degree of rapport is achieved between these two factors, any advertisement of any campaign is doomed to failure.[73]

Quera identifies two barriers standing in the way of success. The first is the volume of advertisements that bombard the target audience every day.

"Any potential consumer faces considerable difficulty in weeding out the message intended solely for him," he says.[74]

The second barrier has to do with the impersonal nature of the media. Quera says:

> While indispensable, media for an advertiser represent an indirect means of presenting reasons for buying his particular product. Objections to buying cannot be overcome immediately as when making a face-to-face sales presentation. With media as a vehicle for advertising, the communicator of a message is placed in a position quite like having to talk through a thick wool blanket.[75]

Quera considers a campaign to be intangible compared to a more concrete advertisement. However, a campaign becomes "the total advertisement in final purpose." He says:

> The advertising question thus becomes not whether or not an advertisement or an advertising campaign will achieve the objectives of expanding sales and increasing profits, but instead which will better gain consumer traffic on a sustained basis. To view the question in this light should result in a conclusion that a campaign of related advertisements will produce more consumer action than individual advertisements issued in isolation.[76]

There also are differences between a "product" and a "service." Quera points out that a product is tangible and can be physically experienced by a consumer while a service has a fundamental intangibility and cannot be physically experienced. These differences carry significant ramifications for formulating an advertising campaign.[77]

Quera says an advertising campaign for a service can include appeals to either rational or emotional buying motives, although emotional is used more often with intangible services. Different media also could be required for different services.[78] Hospitals, for example, might produce their own direct mail magazine, newsletter, or other "personalized" approaches to emphasize a "caring atmosphere" in combination with television and newspaper advertising, which could primarily be used to promote the hospital's advances in research, technology or specialized services. An all-night clinic specializing in pediatrics might choose to advertise on a radio station that appeals to young parents and by placing posters in grocery stores.

Quera emphasizes that all of the ingredients of a marketing mix need to be considered when planning an advertising campaign, but product planning, pricing, branding, channels of distribution, packaging, and promotion are especially important.[79] In addition, every advertising campaign should have a central theme tying together the message of its advertisements. He suggests that "without the formulation of an objective to solve a problem and the design of a strategic approach, the tactic of an advertising campaign is not utilized to fullest potential."[80]

For example, if screening clinics were to be opened in three predominately African American churches, the theme may be something as simple as "be healthy in body and spirit." Various advertisements, then, could first concentrate on the need and convenience for such clinics. The second wave might be more specific about the types of screenings offered. The third wave might attempt to overcome the audience members' fear of disease or specific procedures (needle sticks, for example). The final wave might include testimonials from the local people who received early treatment and/or cures because of the screenings.

The next step is media selection, which Quera considers "one of the more important of many decision to be made in the formulation and tactics of an advertising campaign."[81] He says:

> Among the problems affecting a decision are selection of media by product type, media objectives, comparison of media, and popularity of media class. Added to these are problems of popularity of individual media, size and frequency of advertisements in a campaign, special availabilities and discounts, barter and brokerage, and media selection responsibility.[82]

Because advertising is such an important and expensive portion of the marketing mix, Quera suggests that marketing research to determine advertising effectiveness is imperative. He suggests a review of an advertising program, the type of campaign proposed to carry it out, the theme of the campaign, the selection of media to carry the advertisements of the campaign, and whatever promotion is used to augment the campaign effort followed by subjective and objective approaches to measure the effectiveness of advertisements. These steps can prove more difficult when measuring the effectiveness of a campaign. Measuring the effectiveness of one advertisement, for example, will tell little about the effectiveness of other ads in the campaign. He says:

> While a consumer may remember and react to one particular advertisement of a campaign, more than likely he will be influenced into an actual buying action only after seeing or being exposed to several advertisements of that campaign. As a consequence, the tactic of a campaign normally is more valuable for an advertiser than a single advertisement. As a further consequence, the advertiser customarily is more interested in the effectiveness of the campaign than the effectiveness of the single advertisement.[83]

Although he warns that techniques for measuring the effectiveness of a campaign may be imprecise, Quera suggests that such devices as the test market, advertising budget manipulation, and campaign comparisons should be used to determine when to employ a new advertising campaign.[84]

As Fitzpatrick clearly states:

> The system is largely irrelevant to the fundamental problems of the poor. It meets them in artificial circumstances (the clinic or office), discusses their difficulty in a vocabulary and with a conceptual framework that has no relevance to their total world, and involves them in a treatment process which damages them by labeling them to themselves and their communities. In seeking to treat the mental disorder in isolation from other problems, the system may hopelessly complicate the life of the poor person. Within this process from beginning (diagnosis) to end (treatment), the poor person comes off badly, is unable to protect himself, and sometimes ends up in a worse state than that in which he began.[85]

"The essential power of the poor," as Reissman emphasizes, "has been the veto: to refuse services."[86] Indeed, many African Americans have refused, or at least under-used health care services. It is possible that advertisements for physicians, clinics, and hospitals are meaningless to many African Americans because they do not address the issues that are most important to them. Any information campaign must include specific research to determine the characteristics of the African American population that is targeted, so that advertising principles can be applied and/or altered to better communicate with this population.

Over the past two decades, the mass media have presented an increasing array of health campaigns intended to combat heart disease, cancer, smoking, drug and alcohol abuse, and unsafe driving. Researchers conclude that such campaigns attained only a limited degree of success and identified a key reason: these efforts are underdeveloped at the preparation, production, and dissemination phases of implementation due to poor conceptualization and inadequate evaluation research.

The following discussion will offer solutions to some barriers to implementing an effective information campaign.

COMMUNITY-BASED CAMPAIGNS

Hertog et al. suggest that implementing a community-based public health campaign, another aspect of social marketing, "means more than simply carrying out strategies whose focus is solely individual-level change."[87] They conclude that an individual is less likely to alter his or her behavior in a social environment that is not conducive to change because people do not act as isolated individuals in a social vacuum.

Effective health campaigns must take into consideration community structure and culture:

> In any community, existing lines of power and influence affect both the acceptance of outside influence and the availability of lines of communication within the community. Community leaders can act either to legitimize or delegitimize the actions of health professionals who are attempting to prompt change from the outside. Civic and health leaders within the community are more accepted and trusted by community members due both to experience with the leaders and the feeling of common fate due to the leaders' membership within the community. If the health professional ignores the leadership structure of the community, he/she does so at great risk to the efficacy of the intervention.[88]

They also suggest that existing public health organizations and social and power structures will make some types of intervention far more efficient and effective than others.[89]

To make community health campaigns most effective, the authors suggest first a thorough review of scientific literature concerning public health campaigns, successful and unsuccessful, to guide campaign strategy and to help prevent duplication of earlier mistakes. A thorough review of information concerning the community's structure and public health facilities is valuable, and other areas where information is needed can be identified. Finally, qualitative and quantitative methods should be used to study beliefs, customs, and personal circumstances surrounding health-related behavior.

Once a thorough review of the results of the qualitative analysis has been carried out, the researcher must focus on crucial areas for intervention and test hypotheses concerning these areas and the behavior change advocated. They suggest using large-scale quantitative methods, such as survey research, to determine how certain beliefs and behaviors hang together, defining groups within the population that can be targeted for special messages.[90]

Atkin, Garramone, and Anderson argue that most public service campaigns and health education and persuasion campaigns are created "without sufficient formative evaluation research inputs to guide planning and design," while commercial advertising campaigns are based on "extensive pre-campaign research activities, such as market segmentation analysis, consumer opinion surveys, focus group interviews, and message pretesting."[91] Evaluation research seeks to answer questions about the target audience for a project, program or campaign that includes collection of background information about the orientations of the audience before initiating a campaign, and assessment of the implementation and effectiveness during and after a campaign.[92] They say:

> According to Palmer (1981), *formative research* provides data and perspectives to improve messages during the course of creation. He divides this form of evaluation into two phases; the first involves *preproduction research*, "in which data are accumulated on audience characteristics that relate importantly to the medium, the message, and the situation within which the desired behavior will occur." The second type of formative research is *product testing*, in which prototype or pilot messages are pretested to obtain audience reactions prior to final production.[93]

Instead of systematic approaches, the authors say mass media campaign efforts often proceed in the absence of a research foundation, "produced in a haphazard fashion based on creative inspiration of copywriters and artists, patterned after the normative standards of the health campaign genre."[94] They report that little background information about the audience is used to formulate message appeals and presentation styles, in selecting source spokespersons and channels, or in identifying specialized subgroups to be reached. Also, research is seldom used to set priorities and processes for basic campaign goals and specific objectives.

Atkin, Garramone, and Anderson say the conventional approach to designing communication persuasion strategies involves "dissecting the communication process into source, message, channel, and receiver variables as inputs and a series of information processing and response variables as outcomes."[95] They say a widely used model is McGuire's 1981 input-output matrix, which includes the S-M-C-R variables along with destination factors on the input side of the matrix.[96] The source, channel, and message components are manipulatable by the campaign designer:

> The *source* is generally the visible presenter (rather than the ultimate sponsor or person who constructs the message) from whom the audience perceives the message as coming, who may have varying characteristics in terms of demographics (age, sex, socio-economic status), credibility (expertise, trustworthiness), and attractiveness.
>
> Each *message* can feature a variety of content dimensions (themes, appeals, claims, evidence, and recommendations) using various formats of organization and styles of packaging; the series of messages in a campaign can vary in volume, repetition, prominence of placement, and scheduling.
>
> The *channel* variables comprise both the medium of transmission (television, radio, newspapers, magazines) and the particular media vehicle (e.g., which radio station or magazine title).
>
> *Receiver* factors are not subject to manipulation, but sensitivity to background characteristics, abilities, and predispositions of individuals enhances the effectiveness of campaign stimuli.
>
> Finally, the *destination* label encompasses the array of impacts that the campaign aims to produce, such as immediate vs. long-term change, prevention vs. cessation, direct vs. two-step flow of influence, target variables (including specific behavioral goals and intermediate objectives such as belief formation, attitude change, skills acquisition, and immunization to subsequent counter messages in the interpersonal or media environment), and the size and composition of target segments of the public of primary and secondary priority (e.g., current and potential at-risk subgroups and persons in a position to influence those at risk).[97]

Atkin, Garramone, and Anderson list McGuire's 12 successive response steps as: exposure, attending, liking, comprehending, acquiring skills, yielding, memory storage, retrieval, deciding, behaving, reinforcement and consolidating. However, they say Flay separates the responses into intermediate processes: presentation, attention, comprehension, and acceptance/yielding and dependent variable outcomes: exposure, awareness, knowledge, opinion/belief, attitude, intention, and behavior. Rogers' model of innovation adoption sequence includes: knowledge, persuasion, decision, and confirmation.[98]

Atkin, Garramone, and Anderson combine elements from various models to suggest the following five basic stages, each with several substeps:

> The first is *exposure*, which includes encountering the stimulus and paying attention to it. The next stage is information *processing*, including comprehension of the content, perception of source and appeals, and evaluative reactions such as liking, agreeing, and counterarguing. The third stage is cognitive *learning*, which involves knowledge gain and skills acquisition. Fourth, the *yielding* stage encompasses the formation or change of affective orientations such as beliefs, saliences, values, attitudes, and behavioral intentions. Finally, a *utilization* stage includes retrieval and motivation, the action itself, post-behavioral consolidation, and long-run continuation and maintenance of the practice.[99]

They also say three families of social psychological theories are relevant to health campaigns. These include the instrumental learning perspective used by Hovland, Janis, and Kelley (1953), that focuses attention on factors such as source credibility, the incentives in the message appeal, and repetition; Bandura's (1977) social learning or imitation approach, that emphasizes the importance of the characteristics of source role models, the explicit demonstration of target behaviors, and the depiction of vicarious positive and negative reinforcements; and expectancy-value formulations, particularly the Ajzen and Fishbein (1980) theory of reasoned action, which stresses the role of beliefs concerning the likelihood that performance of a behavior leads to certain consequences, which, when combined with evaluations of the outcomes, determine the attitude.[100]

SOURCE CREDIBILITY

One element of a mass media campaign that often is overlooked, even in social marketing, is source credibility. Rogers and Shoemaker consider credibility to be "the degree to which a communication source or channel is perceived as trustworthy and competent by the receiver."[101] Sharma says that "if an individual perceives a source to possess higher credibility than various other sources, the individual will be more receptive to messages from that source. Credibility is perceived by the receiver and has no objective criteria.[102]

Cognitive response theory, first proposed by Greenwald in 1968, may explain the effect of source credibility. Sharma says:

> The theory suggests that social influence depends on the favorability of thoughts (object-attributions) available in memory at the time of the decision (Harmon and Coney 1982). The two major types of thoughts that buyers will have are message thoughts and own-thoughts. Message thoughts represent the message in the sales presentation and will likely reflect the position of the salesperson. Own-thoughts are object-attributions association stored in the memory relevant to the message being presented.[103]

Further, Sharma says the basic proposition that an individual's attitude change is positively related to the credibility with which he perceives the source of persuasive messages is supported in laboratory experimental studies and survey research in communication.[104] He says:

> The effect of source credibility on attitude and intention depends on whether respondents have expectations or experiences of the product. These initial (pre-contact) expectations are established by the buyers' previous experience with the brand/product/ product-class or based on communication that buyers receive from friends, newspapers, or other salespeople.[105]

If an individual has a negative opinion on an advocacy position, a highly credible source will have a higher level of persuasion and a larger effect on attitude change than a less credible source, Sharma notes. This could be explained by the cognitive response theory, which suggests that when an individual has a negative predisposition toward an issue, a highly credible source will inhibit his or her counter-argumentation which in turn will lead to greater persuasion. Conversely, if an individual has a positive predisposition toward an issue, a less credible source will increase support arguments, which leads to greater persuasion. An increase in support arguments occurs when individuals have a positive predisposition toward an issue or they feel the need to ensure that the position to which they agree is adequately represented, but when individuals have a positive pre-disposition toward an issue, a highly credible source does not increase support arguments and is not as persuasive as a less credible source.[106]

This suggests that source credibility should also be tested when planning a campaign. Not only should the credibility of the campaign sponsor (state health department, local hospital or clinic, or community coalition), but any spokesperson used in advertising or in promotion should also be tested.

For example, focus group discussions used for this research indicated that African Americans may not want a physician dictating behavior changes to them. Consequently, a community leader such as a minister or politician might be received more favorably than a physician. Likewise, care must be exercised in selecting a prominent person to be a spokesperson for a campaign. Although the members of the focus group indicated they enjoyed hearing or reading about African American entertainers, athletes and others who have "achieved" something in life, such heroes can fall from grace quickly (e.g., Michael Jackson, Magic Johnson, O.J. Simpson) and can do more harm than good.

The most credible source may be someone from the community with whom the audience members can identify and who they believe will have no ulterior motive in promoting the health campaign. There was a feeling in one focus group conducted for this study that a white spokesperson does not carry the weight of a black spokesperson when diseases that are especially prevalent in the black population are the focus of an advertisement or a campaign. However, a multi-cultural approach (for example, having a prominent black minister and a prominent white minister presented together) might be very effective.

It also seems likely that a federal government program might not have the same level of credibility as a local program simply because there may be more distrust of large, tax-supported projects than smaller community projects that can be made more tangible. However, a local program combined with a federal program may bolster credibility over all. The point is, it is important to determine the source credibility of those involved in a campaign as early as possible.

TARGETING AUDIENCES

Atkin, Garramone, and Anderson advocate preproduction research, which is formulated to learn as much as possible about the target audience "before specifying goals and devising strategies to locate audience segments and move them through the appropriate stages of response to campaign stimuli."[107] The objective should be to identify the demographic and psychographic characteristics of the audience and to determine channel usage patterns. In addition, the audience's current communication patterns, cognitions, affective orientations, and behaviors pertaining to the subject of the campaign should be determined. They also say:

> Topic-specific information is sought concerning the audience's current communication patterns, cognitions, affective orientations, and behaviors pertaining to the subject of the campaign: prior media exposure to messages relating to the topic (ads, PSA's, news, features, entertainment) and reactions to such content, interpersonal communication (contact with topical opinion leaders, discussion of topic, exposure to personal influence), entry level knowledge (awareness and information-holding about subject: what is known, what gaps exist, what misinformation exists), beliefs and images (subjective conceptions of the topic already held, particularly the estimated probabilities of outcomes associated with behaviors and perceived social norms), values and attitudes (desirability of outcomes, evaluations of concepts related to topic), salience levels (perceived importance of objects and attributes involving topic), personal efficacy (subjective competency to carry out actions), and behavior patterns (frequency of actions, situational behavioral tendencies). For some specialized topics or audiences, background information may be needed about abilities (general intellectual development, basic cognitive capacity, degree of sophistication) and lexicon (understanding of vocabulary and terminology relevant to subject-matter). Furthermore, campaigners need to ascertain audience responsiveness to various dimensions of potential campaign stimuli (receptivity to concept ideas, perceived credibility of source presenters, preferences among stylistic approaches).[108]

Manoff points out that target audience identification involves a variety of factors such as health, economics, life-style, convenience, and image. He says identifying these factors is necessary to differentiate targets if sharply focused message and media strategies are to be devised.[109]

Grunig emphasizes that new studies show information campaigns are more likely to succeed when they are aimed at "carefully selected segments of the mass audience."[110] He says the basic idea of segmentation is to divide a population, market, or audience into groups whose members are more like each other than members of other segments based on demographics, psychographics, values and lifestyles, geodemographic clusters of postal zip codes, geographic regions, consumer behaviors, elasticities of consumer responses to products, product benefits, amount of consumption, and purchase/use situations.[111]

Audience segments, Grunig says, must be "definable, mutually exclusive, measurable, accessible, pertinent to an organization's mission, reachable with communications in an affordable way, and large enough to be substantial and to service economically."[112] He acknowledges that market segments may meet these criteria but still respond in similar fashions to a communication strategy. Consequently, segments need not be isolated and defined unless they respond differently to an information campaign. He says:

> When marketing theorists use the term *differential response,* their unspoken assumption is that the desired response is behavioral: a purchase, adoption, use or similar desired behavior. . . . . (H)owever, communication campaigns—including marketing communication campaigns—cannot always be evaluated by monitoring behavioral responses. Behaviors usually are less sensitive to campaigns than are variables that occur earlier in the behavioral chain that begins with seeking of or exposure to a message and continues through cognition, attitude, and behavior.[113]

Grunig argues that campaigns need not always target behavior changes. He says they also may seek to affect cognition (e.g., accuracy and understanding) and attitudes either to have "an intermediary effect on the path to individual or collective behavioral change" or as ends in themselves. Also, it may be possible to "affect collective behavior by creating and mobilizing activist, issue groups."[114]

Grunig advocates the reliance on a "nested approach" to segment audiences. The basic idea is that it may be necessary to targeted easily identifiable groups in order to reach the smaller, more subtle and hard-to-assess segments included within the groups. He explains the layers of nests in this way:

> The innermost nest contains variables that predict *individual communication behaviors and effects*—the perfect concepts for segmentation if it were feasible to organize campaigns for individuals. The second nest defines *publics*—individuals who communicate and behave in similar ways. For most campaigns, publics represent the optimal segment, optimal because that segment maximizes the differential responses desired by campaign planners at a reasonable cost. These first two nests are related, however, because one must understand the behaviors of individuals to understand the behaviors of publics.[115]

Subsequent nests, Grunig says, consist of *communities; psychographics, lifestyles, subcultures, and social relationships; geodemographics; demographics and social categories;* and, finally, *mass audiences.* He concludes:

> A variable in an inner nest can pinpoint a public or a market segment precisely. A variable in an outer nest can locate the segments in the inner nests, also, although it will not be able to discriminate among several segments that could be identified by variables in the inner nest. . . . The groupings in the outer nests are less powerful in isolating communication behaviors and effects than are those in the two inner nests. The outer nests may contain the publics that are the segment targeted by a communication campaign, but they also contain publics that are not targeted.[116]

Segmentation may be most easily accomplished by starting with the inner nests and working outward, although the amount of funding available for a campaign may dictate the opposite, less expensive route. The community nest may overlap both the public nest within it and the lifestyles nest above it, because members of publics may be found in several communities, and several lifestyles may be found in the same community.[117]

Grunig next addresses the "problem" of determining whether the audience in the innermost nest is active or passive. He points out that the uses and gratifications theory (described in Chapter III) assumes an active audience. However, critics of this theory (e.g., Carey and Kreiling, 1974; Biocca, 1988) argue that media use "is more passive, consummatory, and under the control of the media rather than the audience." Grunig's solution to this dilemma is that communication behavior can be either active or passive.[118] He admits, however, that the crucial theoretical problem is to find concepts that predict the circumstances under which communication behavior is active or passive. Determining the "social and psychological origins" of the "needs" that supposedly motivate human communication is an area which he believes needs further exploration.

In the meantime, Grunig suggests focusing on needs, problems, situations, and issues to segment the audience in the innermost nest. He relies on Assael's definition of *needs* as "inner motivational states that are aroused by external stimuli or internal cues,"[119] which Grunig suggests implies people cannot control their behavior. His view is that people can control their behavior, although they do not in some situations. The characteristics of these situations can be identified. Using *problems*, rather than *needs*, is easier for the researcher because understanding that "problem recognition motivates communication behavior, researchers can ask people what problems they recognize to determine what they will communicate about and whether they will respond to a communication campaign about particular topics."[120]

Grunig says marketing researchers have used situations, such as physical and social surroundings, time, the specific task for which a product is used, personal state-of-mind at purchase, social or financial pressure, uncertainty, or a situation served inadequately by existing products as methods of audience segmentation.[121] Finally, Grunig relates *issues* to the agenda-setting approach (described in Chapter III) to mass media effects because audience members may use issues as means of processing news.[122]

Regarding the next nest—publics—Grunig says:

> Although the variables identified in the first nest could allow planners to target individuals for communication campaigns, such microsegmentation is seldom possible—even when interpersonal communication is a primary vehicle for the campaign. Publics, in the second nest, therefore, represent the first level of aggregation necessary for a campaign. It is a useful level of aggregation, however, because it allows researchers to place individuals into groups that differ in the extent to which they actively communicate, construct cognition and attitudes, and engage in individual or collective behaviors—the primary differential responses sought from a campaign.[123]

Grunig says marketing theorists most often refer to segments as markets, but public relations theorists call these segments *publics*. He argues that although target segments for public communication campaigns may be either publics or markets, publics are usually more active than markets. His distinction between a market and a public is that the two inner nests describe publics, whereas the outer nests describe markets. He concludes that public relations practitioners more often use inner nests for segmentation, while marketing practitioners use the outer nests.[124]

Grunig groups psychographics, lifestyles, subcultures, and social relationships into one nest because they represent population segments grouped by psychological or social characteristics, or both. To segment at this level, Grunig recommends psychographic techniques such as VALS (for values and lifestyles) or AIO items (for activities, interests, and opinions).[125] These are advertising and marketing concepts that were developed primarily to aggregate consumers into likely buying groups. For example, a "high tech" group might consist of people with home computers and VCRs. They would be likely consumer targets for compact disc players, satellite dishes, and other new electronic devices. Likewise, people who enjoy sports and exercising could be targeted for fitness equipment.

Subcultures, Grunig says, are narrower than national cultures and consist of people with similar values, customs, norms, beliefs, and behaviors.[126]

Grunig believes social relationships are important in explaining how people use media and how the media affect them. He says:

> To be useful in segmentation, the concept of social relationships must be converted into measurable variables. The concepts . . . (of) psychographics, lifestyles, and culture, provide the variables and the measures needed to convert the idea of social relationships into measured segments.[127]

Grunig draws on diffusion of innovations theory (described in Chapter III) to augment segmentation in this nest. He says the most important contribution that diffusion theory makes to the nested model is its identification of characteristics of adopter categories (especially social relationships) that fall into outer nests.[128]

Hornik says that network studies are strong evidence that social relationships play a major part in diffusion of information and practice, although he questions whether any study has shown that networks mediate the effects of mass communication. He says:

> In order to show that the effects of mass communication are different depending on the social networks in which an individual is embedded, one has to be able to contrast networks that vary in their support of the message transmitted through public information channels. One needs to show that if a network is supportive, knowledge (garnered from a public information campaign) turns into behavior and that if the network is unsupportive, individuals are less likely to turn knowledge into behavior.[129]

Grunig's geodemographic nest contains a segmentation technique widely used in marketing and public relations that consists partly of lifestyles and partly of geographic demographics. He says:

> Geodemographic segmentation, lifestyle segmentation, suffers because it falls in an outer nest and does not predict communication behavior and the existence of publics directly. Planners of communication programs can purchase geodemographic data easily, however, and these data can provide a reasonable substitute for original research to identify publics.[130]

Grunig advocates the use of demographics "to avoid unfocused dissemination of information to a mass audience, in part because demographics help to explain use of different media." He says demographics also serve as useful locators of publics and other segments in inner nests, although he warns that the segments identified by demographics usually do not overlap publics closely. Demographics may be the only segmentation tool available to the communication planner, Grunig acknowledges, because time and/or money may not permit other research. [131]

Concerning his final nest, Grunig says that communication campaigns will seldom be effective if they are directed to a mass audience. Although mass audiences do have segments embedded in them that communicate actively and messages directed at an unsegmented population may reach the active segments, the costs of the this type of campaign will be much greater than campaigns using other nests.[132]

Atkin, Garramone, and Anderson point out that various research techniques are available to obtain the types of information mentioned above. These techniques include survey research using sampling frames, focus groups, in-depth interviews, and data bases such as Arbitron or Nielsen ratings, readership studies, and demographic profiles.[133]

MESSAGES

Message content is of special interest to those engaged in social marketing. The previous discussion shows how audiences can be segmented. This section will discuss elements that contribute to an effective message.

Wilde offers advice about how to create effective messages. He says effectiveness depends upon the opinion the receiver holds toward the source. Affecting this opinion are the source's perceived credibility, expertise, trustworthiness, and similarity with the recipient.[134]

According to Manoff, typical prevention messages are simple and direct—demanding little technical preparation. He says they depend as much on emotive, persuasive power as on information. They should be directed to behavioral and life-style traits of the affluent as well as to the special concerns of the less fortunate.

Flay and Burton contend that the content of the message and the quality of its production will be considered by media gatekeepers. They warn:

> The content cannot be too controversial for most gatekeepers, nor be seen
> as possibly evoking other controversial issues. . . . Production quality must
> be similar to other material used by the chosen channel.[135]

In addition the message and its source and the channel used to distribute it must be acceptable to the target audience and effective at influencing them. Flay and Burton argue that only influential messages from believable sources will change people or society, regardless of how many people are reached on how many occasions.[136]

Flay and Burton identify three major areas—needs assessment, application of theory, and formative research—that can influence high-quality messages, sources, and channels. Needs assessment includes identifying the problem, knowing the target audience, and knowing the relevant societal conditions surrounding the issue and social attitudes toward it. Application of theory involves message content and structure, knowledge of the target audience, and the general structure of the campaign. Formative research implies concepts and preproduction messages should be pretested with samples of the target audience before final production. To be effective, a message must reach the target audience, be repeated frequently and consistently but with some novelty, for long periods of time.[137]

Devine and Hirt say the primary difference between message-based and behavioral- based persuasion centers around the source of initial information that provides the basis for the attitude (i.e., either a message from a communicator or the recipient's own experience). They argue:

> These persuasion strategies may be differentially appropriate to certain types of situations, issues and/or desired outcomes. For instance, under conditions in which people are sufficiently motivated to carefully attend to and evaluate the communication (i.e., conditions of high personal relevance), message-based persuasion may be the most appropriate strategy. If message arguments are strong (i.e., cogent, well-reasoned), persuasion is likely to occur. However, under conditions of low personal relevance, behavior-based persuasion may be most effective. For example, in an advertising situations in which consumers need to make decisions among essentially equivalent products, . . . inducing the consumer to try the product may provide the most compelling information about the product. Given a favorable experience with the product, the consumer may then be willing to purchase the product again, potentially leading to the development of commitment or brand loyalty. Message-based strategies would be hard-pressed to develop convincing arguments that would sufficiently differentiate among the products.[138]

Grunig, in considering the implications of the social psychological literature for information campaigns, also draws a distinction between message-based persuasion and behavioral persuasion. He says the goal for both types is to influence attitudes that are assumed to guide behavior with respect to the attitude object. He says, therefore:

> Message-based persuasion, which is dependent on providing audience members with a message and arguments to support the message, would be most effective under conditions in which (1) mass media are available and affordable, (2) there is little opportunity for interpersonal contact among campaigners and the target audience, (3) the campaign conveys a compelling and understandable message, (4) the audience has at least some general familiarity with the topic (e.g., issue, product, social policy) of the campaign, and (5) the goal is to produce repeated behaviors.

Behavioral-based persuasion strategies, on the other hand, seem to be better suited to situations in which (1) mass media presentation of messages is limited; (2) there are opportunities for interpersonal contact that may allow campaigners to take advantage of some of the heuristic (e.g., reciprocity) processes summarized previously; (3) there is little difference among response alternatives (e.g., laundry detergents); (4) the audience is unfamiliar with the attributes of the topic of the campaign (e.g., issue, product, social policy); (5) the goal is to produce one-time and/or repeated behaviors. . . .[139]

He points out that neither strategy is better than the other, and that, when resources are available, a blend of message-based and behavioral-based persuasion is the ideal strategy.

MEDIA SELECTION

Once messages have been devised and tested, the next logical step is to identify dissemination methods. Among the most pervasive and powerful channels are the mass media. Researchers have examined the role the mass media plays in information campaigns.

Atkin and Arkin say "the evolving relationship between the mass communication and public health sectors is played out in the context of a rapidly changing media and regulatory environment."[140] They identify four trends that contribute to this relationship: diversification of the media; increasing public interest in health information; and the Reagan administration's era of deregulation, resulting in less public service time for public health messages and less oversight of health-related portrayals and advertising claims by severely trimmed network "standards and practices" departments.[141] They say:

At least one-forth of all articles in daily newspapers are in some way related to health, yet some stories that are considered important by the public health community receive little or no coverage. There is a basic conflict between what gatekeepers judge to be newsworthy and what health specialists believe the public should be told. Basically, the public health community wants positive coverage, it wants its messages used intact, it wants coverage that explains the complexities and uncertainties of science, and it wants illumination of structural-risk factors, rather than a focus on individuals with health problems.[142]

Manoff argues that much of the research in health education mass media campaigns is based on questionable assumptions:

> *Questionable Assumption #1. The mass media are monoliths and their impact is measurable without recourse to evaluation of message design, the length of the media schedule (continuity), or the frequency of exposure (media weight).* Until they are given a message to deliver and a schedule to manage its delivery, the mass media are neutral entities. It is the message, combined with media weight and continuity, that determines media effectiveness, not vice versa.
>
> *Questionable Assumption #2. Messages have a uniform value entirely dependent on media effectiveness for their impact.* This is the converse of QA#1 and is invalid for the same reasons.
>
> *Questionable Assumption #3. The duration of mass media campaigns is immaterial to their effectiveness. . . .* For the most part the typical evaluation disregards significant differences in media weight, reach, frequency, and continuity and confines itself to measuring impact on the target audience, which cannot be meaningfully interpreted without evaluation of these values. A true evaluation analyzes the process, assessing the relationship of all parts to the whole; it cannot merely be an audit for results with no insight into what was right or wrong. . . .
>
> *Questionable Assumption #4. There is no qualitative difference among the mass media in terms of potential impact on the target audience.* Mass media projects are frequently imprecise in the selection of media and undiscriminating in their categorization. Leaflets, posters, and films are often classified as mass media along with radio and TV, and this indifference to comparative media values is reciprocated in the typical evaluation. . . .
>
> *Questionable Assumption #5. Radio, TV, newspaper, and magazine exposure is a gross quantity unaffected by channel selection and program adjacencies on radio and TV or by the choice of publications and the positions messages are assigned in them.* The assurance that messages will be efficiently delivered to their target populations obliges the health educator to identify the stations, programs and the print-media sections with the highest concentration of desired viewers, listeners, or readers. . . .[143]

Conversely, Manoff offers some safe assumptions about the mass media:

Mass media assure thorough control of the message.
Mass media lend a cumulative impact to the message.
Mass media reach the masses.
Mass media telescope time.
Mass media influence other major audiences in important ways while directing a message to its target audience.
The mass media campaign enhances the effectiveness of all other methods employed in health education.[144]

There also are studies that suggest the media try to preserve the status quo. Shoemaker, for example, has found that newspaper editors are more receptive to information from groups they perceived as legitimate, viable, and centrist (e.g., the League of Women Voters) than from groups perceived as lacking those characteristics (e.g., the Jewish Defense League or the Nazi Party).[145]

Meyer takes another approach. He emphasizes the media are a market that must be understood by anyone who wants to use them. To the textbook definition of news values—timeliness, proximity, consequence, human interest, conflict, prominence, and unusualness—Meyer adds the following:

Inoffensiveness. Editors protect the sensibilities of their readers, reminding each other that a newspaper is a family medium.
The window of credibility. If an event is unusual, that helps it to qualify as news up to a point. Beyond that point, its unusualness creates such a strain on the belief system of the audience that it will not be attended to.
Fitting existing constructs. To avoid information overload, we perceive the world in terms of types and generalities—stereotypes. Collections of stereotypes form constructs or theoretical models through which we interpret the busy flow of facts and images. To qualify as news, an account must fit the prevailing constructs.
Packageable in daily bites. Competition and the daily cycle require news to be shaped into small, discrete packages, even when the events it describes may not be easily adaptable to that form.[146]

This discussion of the media are included because social marketing assumes that the mass media is a vital and powerful tool in information campaigns. However, campaign planners must understand the barriers that may prevent effective use of the media. In other words, planners of a health campaign should not assume that the mainstream media will be receptive to and supportive of their efforts. In fact, campaigns that target minority groups, such as African Americans—may find the media disinterested because editors and reporters may assume that only a small segment of their audience will be interested in the topic. It is imperative that campaign planners know the media's biases and constraints in order to counteract them. Also, media that cater to African Americans, such as black newspapers, magazines, and radio stations, should be used to the fullest extent possible. They have many of the restraints associated with the mainstream media, but they are much more likely to be aware of and concerned about problems affecting the black community.

COMMUNITY-BASED CAMPAIGNS

Social marketing recognizes the importance of "getting to know" target communities in as much detail as possible. Finnegan, Bracht, and Viswanath say the rationale underlying community-based campaigns is that "social and cultural influences are crucial factors in learning and adopting behavior patterns and importantly, that these influences are experienced by individuals through social aggregates and networks that make up communities."[147]

They point out that many community-based campaigns have been stimulated in part by developing interdisciplinary theories about ways to solve social problems and to improve the quality of life often with the goal of bringing about changes in health care behavior. These types of campaigns differ from other kinds of campaigns "by seeking complex, long-term outcomes, often in several related behavioral areas defined as 'lifestyle,' (daily living and work habits); by the use of multiple strategies for intervention, and by an emphasis on 'community' as the nexus of social relations which form individual behavior."[148]

Finnegan et al. say one of the most important dimensions of community-based campaigns is their emphasis on mobilizing whole communities as an overall strategy to enhance the potential for individuals to change.[149] They say three themes unify these views about the process of seeking long-term social and behavior change:

> First is the emphasis on powerful social forces influencing individuals' behavior—the idea that behavior is formed and influenced by the dominant culture and individuals' social relations in the context of their communities. . . .

A second common theme is that communities themselves may be mobilized to act as change agents to achieve social and behavioral outcomes. . . . Practically, mobilizing communities means engaging networks of public and private organizations and special interest groups to channel their resources . . . in coordinated activity in a broad range of interpersonal, group and mass communication strategies. . . . [150]

They add that legitimacy is particularly important to community-based campaigns:

(Legitimacy) is the process through which social leaders "give sanction, justification, (and) the license to act," influencing the rest of the community to adopt desired changes. But an equally important tangible outcome is that groups with power to allocate resources may change their capacity to provide opportunities for individuals to engage in behavior-change activity . . . . [151]

Their third theme stresses that campaign planning needs to be systematic and data-based, not only to identify traditional audience, source, message and channel variables, but also to identify specific powerful individuals and groups who may mobilize their support and resources to act as change agents.[152]

The authors suggest that space, social institutions, social interaction, and social control are important in the formation of strategies. They add that some key characteristics on which communities may be compared and contrasted are: complexity, linkage and relationships, power and influence, dependence-autonomy and formality, community identify, and social integration.[153]

Obviously, in planning a health care campaign aimed at African Americans it is important to determine geographic area, but even more important to examine the social structure (clubs and organizations), the power structure (influential politicians, ministers, and educators), and the "personality" (civic pride, level of integration, etc.) of the target community or communities. Messages should be developed, media should be selected, and collaboration should be established in conjunction with the community identity.

EVALUATING CAMPAIGN EFFECTIVENESS

In spite of the obvious need to determine whether a campaign has achieved some or all of its goals, many planners fail to do any evaluation or they measure the wrong variables. This is most likely due to lack of funding (evaluation research is often expensive) or the lack of expertise (using ineffective or inconclusive research methods). As Salmon cautions:

> . . . the search for a definitive answer to the question, "Are campaigns effective?" is a search for a minotaur, as the functions, durations, potentials, and levels of creativity and resources are exceptionally heterogeneous. Further, because we have often tended to focus on the "trees," that is, those discrete, obvious, visible and often short-term mass media efforts aimed at the general population, we have tended to ignore the "forest," that is, those pervasive yet disguised long-term efforts aimed at legislative bodies as well as citizens and conducted by literally hundreds of trade associations, governments (foreign and domestic), and interest impact of campaigns on the nexus of social values and institutions that comprise the social context of campaigns.

Mirroring this diversity in campaign composition, duration and intensity is similar diversity in criteria for success. Historically, evaluation of campaigns have consisted of examinations of *effectiveness* rather than *effects*, with the former term referring to those outcomes unexpected or unintended outcomes. [154]

Devine and Hirt begin at the beginning by saying that unless a campaign has clear goals from the start, it is impossible to ascertain what would be appropriate and valid measures of campaign effectiveness. They say:

> . . . we argue that even if the central issue for campaigners is to obtain a specific outcome—whether it be knowledge, attitudes, or behavior—the key to successful campaigns is an understanding of the processes that lead to that outcome . . . an understanding of persuasion as a process allows campaign planners to expeditiously design message strategies to achieve desired goals. In the absence of this understanding, campaigners may use inappropriate or inefficient strategies or strategies needlessly targeted at a secondary rather than a primary goal of most campaigns—namely, human behavior. [155]

They maintain that "most theories of persuasion operate under the assumption that producing attitude change is the key to producing behavior change" and that "some persuasion strategies try to affect attitudes directly through message factors, whereas other strategies attempt to influence attitudes indirectly through behavior."[156]

Grunig says social psychology has provided a number of suggestions to improve the measurement of campaign effectiveness. He agrees that the most effective measures are tied to goal identification:

> If the goal identified is global, then campaigners would be wise to measure a broad range of campaign-relevant behaviors if they are to fully measure campaign effectiveness. Otherwise, they may conclude that a campaign has not been effective when, in reality, they simply failed to measure the right behavior(s). In addition, the social psychological literature would encourage campaigners to measure such behaviors (or attitudes or information) over time when the goal is to produce long-term changes. The decision of when to assess effectiveness appears to be somewhat arbitrary, and campaigners may "miss" the changes produced.[157]

Grunig says the ultimate goal in most information campaigns is to produce campaign-consistent behaviors, and, as such, behavior change is crucial for the success of campaigns.

Social psychologists have identified several factors that increase attitude-behavior consistency (e.g., direct experience, vested interest, confidence, low self-monitoring), and Grunig suggests that a variety of other techniques (e.g., self-prediction, imagination, and role playing) could contribute to improving the attitude-behavior relation. He says recent advances in the attitude-behavior connection, used in conjunction with message-based and behavioral-based persuasion, can help to increase the likelihood of successful campaigns.[158]

Manoff suggests social marketing message cannot be designed without up front research of target audiences' perceptions of problems and solutions. He says:

> Academicians know such research as formative evaluation, the procedure to help form the activity and provide the baseline. This is distinct from summative evaluation or data gathering for evaluation. The techniques may be qualitative or quantitative or a combination of the two. But the

need to understand the workings of the human mind makes qualitative research invaluable to the social marketer.[159]

Manoff points out that most research attempting to assess the real influence of the mass media on behavioral change has proved inconclusive. He says the information- processing research model has been confined to measuring the impact on knowledge, attitude, and behavior of the medium, assuming that message's design quality has a fixed value and is not also a variable to be measured. He concludes that "when evaluation reveals little or no impact from a mass media project or the results are indecisive, the conclusion invariably is that the medium has failed to fulfill its purpose."[160]

However, he argues that failure may lie more with ineptly designed message that misidentify the target audience; are insensitive to cultural considerations; or fail to deal effectively with audience resistance points or to have identified those points in advance, internal message dissonances, and problems of clarity or comprehension. He also argues the media plan may be at fault through inappropriate media selection for the target audience or the message, inadequate media exposure, or media mix. Further, he says "mass media impact is determined by message quality and the exposure the message is given in terms of audience focus and reach and frequency of delivery." [161]

Atkin and Arkin are concerned with audience characteristics. They say:

> Although there is a great deal of media content conveying health care information and persuasion, it is apparent that people pay attention to a relatively small proportion of available material. This exposure barrier is especially a problem for news and public service messages, which are largely ignored or avoided by many segments of the population. Researchers should explore the range of needs, interests, and tastes that motive individuals to select health care messages encountered in the media, and identify the reasons for nonexposure or inattentiveness. . . .[162]

In assessing the actual impact of a campaign, diverse outcome variables can be measured beyond the standard criteria of awareness and attitude change. Atkin and Arkin say:

> . . . At the cognitive level, researchers should examine the acquisition of applied knowledge that is relevant to the individual's personal health care

situation (e.g., learning useful information to cope with a problem), the formation of mental images of health care-related concepts, objects, and roles (e.g., products, life-styles, victims, or care providers), the development of perceptions about real-world phenomena (e.g. perceived prevalence of certain practices or diseases, or conceptions about the social and economic origins of public health care problems), the creation of personal beliefs about the consequences of health care-related behaviors (e.g., risk probabilities), and alterations in agenda salience levels (e.g., relative significance of various public health care problems facing society, or importance of certain consequences of behaviors).

At the affective level, researchers can measure interest in health care subjects, preferences among health care-related products, and critical evaluation skills for processing health care claims and portrayals. Besides attitudinal conversion, investigations can also examine the creation, reinforcement, and maintenance of attitudes, opinions, and values (e.g., forming an opinion on a new health care issue, strengthening an existing attitude, or preserving a health carey value in the face of social pressures).[163]

Because fundamental health care practices are unlikely to change dramatically in response to a single media stimulus, Atkin and Arkin argue "there is a need for measurement that uses highly sensitive scaling or that assesses cumulative impact over a long period of exposure to multiple messages." Also, behaviors beyond personal practices, such as interpersonal discussion of health care topics and social interventions to influence the actions of other people, should be examined.[164]

They also believe researchers should broaden the scope of analysis to include "higher-order aggregations (e.g., impact on couples, families, groups, organizations, and communities) and differential responses across segments of the population (e.g., social categories based on age, gender, race, social class, and health care status)." This type of research provides "ecologically valid assessment of media influence and permits specification of the unequal distribution of effects among subgroups (e.g., knowledge gaps due to differences in health care message access, exposure, processing, or learning)."[165]

Flay and Burton focus on the effects of mass media communication. They believe mass media campaigns can raise awareness and increase knowledge; although attitude change and motivation to act differently are harder to accomplish and substantial behavior change is even more difficult, but not impossible. They rely on social learning theory (Bandura, 1977, 1986) and the health care belief model (Becker, 1974), among other theories, to suggest that behavior change can be accomplished. The following suggestions are consistent not only with basic behavior change theory, but also with increasing attention, interpersonal communication, social support, and reinforcement of change:

1. Demonstrate or model the desired behavior.
2. Present the behavior as effective in achieving desirable objectives, particularly immediate ones such as feeling and looking better.
3. Present the behavior as pertinent to real-life circumstances, rather than in the abstract. Heighten the incentive or value of a particular level of freedom from risk.
4. Instill the belief that a particular act or pattern of behavior will preclude or ameliorate a specific risk. Nurture the motive to avoid harm or improve well-being in the longer term.
5. Present the behavior as enjoying the approval and support of the community.
6. Mobilize public support for the desired changes.
7. Provide specific guidance for the self-management of behavior change.
8. Provide specific guidance for the self-management of relapses by recycling and trying again.
9. Encourage the development of interpersonal social support for change attempts and changed behavior.
10. Provide the infrastructures to support change attempts and changed behavior, encouraging the use of existing infrastructures, or encouraging proactive behavior by the target audience to apply pressure on government or other responsible agencies to provide such infrastructures.
11. Encourage activism against any part of the social system that tends to undermine the desired behavioral changes.[166]

While formative research is useful in assessing the initial variables that likely will affect the success of a campaign, summative evaluation can assist in determining the effects of a particular campaign. Flay and Burton discuss three broad models of evaluation of single studies and synthesis approach:

The *advertising model* focuses on the beginning of the presumed causal chain; it is usually limited to assessing total audience size and recall and recognition of the message. The *impact monitoring model* focuses near the end of the presumed causal chain, using archival data. The use of per capita consumption of tobacco to determine the effects of counteradvertising and publicity is probably the best example of this approach. . . . The *experimental model* attempts a more comprehensive assessment of effects from different levels of the presumed causal chain, and it also attempts to control for alternative explanations for any observed effects. It is the model most favored by scholars, but the one most difficult to implement in the real world.[167]

Flay and Burton conclude that seven implications for campaign design can be drawn from the exploration of theory and practice:

1. It is desirable to meet every one of the conditions discussed; indeed, most of them are necessary. . . .
2. One clear implication is the need for more research at the front end of the campaign design, particularly needs assessment and formative research. . . .
3. Planners should pay greater attention to dissemination. . . .
4. Audience attention, acceptance, and change can be maximized by careful work at all the earlier steps in production. . . .
5. Campaign designers should also maximize favorable interpersonal communication about the campaign issue, particularly among members of the target audience.
6. Planners should always aim for both individual and societal level changes rather than confining themselves to one level or the other.
7. Some type of summative evaluation should always be conducted so the public health care community can learn to do better in the future.[168]

Information campaigns, especially those using social marketing methods, require evaluative research at every step of the process. To design a campaign aimed at African Americans it is necessary to determine audience, message, and media characteristics. At various intervals throughout the duration of the campaign, the effectiveness of the message, distribution methods, and initial audience reactions should be assessed. Finally, once the campaign is completed or is ready to move to a new level, summative research should be undertaken to evaluate the overall impact of the campaign, assessing opinion, knowledge, attitude, and behavior changes. These types of research, of course, require a great deal of funding and commitment from those conducting the campaign. This chapter concludes with a summary of some health care campaigns that have been determined to be successful. The concluding chapters of this book demonstrate methods to obtain formative research on audience characteristics (demographics and psychographics determined through survey research and focus groups) and audience segmentation and message formulation techniques (Q methodology, factor analysis, and telephone survey methods) in order to devise a health care campaign aimed at African Americans.

POTENTIAL CAMPAIGN FOCUSES

The final installment of Eric Adler's four-part series on African American health care in Kansas City, Mo., lists several problems, many related to habits and attitudes, that could be addressed by a health care care campaign. One is diet. Dr. Jasper Fullard Jr., president of the Black Health Care Coalition in Kansas City emphasized that "soul food" is literally killing African Americans in Kansas City. "We as blacks must understand why we are dying early!" Fullard says. "The salt we use. The fat. The cholesterol in our food."[169]

The article also points out that alcohol and tobacco consumption are major problems facing the black community, so teaching people to ignore advertisements, billboards, and commercials aimed at black consumers and romanticize these products is one possible way to try to change attitudes and behaviors. Heatlh care officials are frustrated with media and advertisers who promote alcohol and tobacco on billboards in high numbers in the inner city and present few role models for blacks to promote health carey living.

"There have to be better efforts from all media to combat this problem," Fullard says. "When it comes to positive images we're left out." Additionally, television commercials promoting health carey lifestyles usually feature white actors, making it harder for black consumers to relate to the messages, Adler writes.[170]

The health care officials interviewed also advocate the promotion of exercise, safe sex and non-violence and the counteracting of a cultural philosophy called "fatalism." Dr. Mark Mitchell, formerly Kansas City's minority specialist in the Missouri Department of Heatlh Care, defines fatalism as a pervasive and insidious attitude that began gripping black Americans generations ago. It's an attitude that says, "Why not drink, smoke or use drugs?" because what hope is there of rising above poverty, avoiding teen-age pregnancy or escaping violence?[171]

Heatlh care officials say the media constantly reinforced fatalism by depicting black Kansas Citians as either victims or criminals and generally, as a poverty-stricken and disenfranchised part of society. "If you live in the ghetto and areas that are depressed, your concept of life is depressed," Fullard says. "That's a concept we have to change. And that's not easy."[172]

William Mayfield, regional minority health care coordinator for the U.S. Public Heatlh care Service in Kansas City, says, "You're talking about changing people's lifestyles, their cultural habits. But people in the community have to take some of the responsibilities. You have to take responsibility and initiative to improve your own health care."[173]

The black community has taken several steps to intervene in the cycle of fatalism. The Black Health Care Coalition, for example, has obtained funding for informational materials, health care fairs, and clinics set up in five black churches to screen for high blood pressure, diabetes and high cholesterol levels. In addition to the clinics, black churches and community clinics have sponsored youth groups and other health care-related activities to try to instill preventive measures, including changing diet, using birth control and curbing aggressive behavior.

The total efforts of these grassroots campaigns are to build positive self-images and to try to promote the sense that it is important to be healthy both for yourself and for your family or those depending on you. "The idea is to give people something to look forward to, something to strive for," Fullard says.[174]

THE VERGENT REPORT

Somewhat ironically, Stephenson researched many of the health care concerns of African Americans in Kansas City, Mo., in the 1960s. His main goal was to increase participation in what was then the Wayne Miner Neighborhood Heatlh Care Center (now the Samuel Rogers Heatlh Care Center). He and a team of researchers (many were his students) examined values, attitudes, and opinions of those who would most benefit from the

Center and formulated pamphlets and films based on Stephenson's theories of communication and advertising. Stephenson summarizes the research he and his students completed in the Vergent Report as follows:

> It is widely held, to judge by the universality of its practice, that if only we could *inform* people about medical matters they would take notice and do what is necessary about them. Efforts are made to make the information interesting, with lively copy, fine photography, expert typography, first-class film direction and production and the like: our studies show, however, that all of this is to no avail unless and until the intended audiences are studied, and their interests understood. For it is amongst the first laws of communication that audiences only really attend to what interests them in a personal sense—it is not an interesting film or pamphlet *per se*, but an *interest in the person* to which the pamphlet makes its ploy. A person ill with cancer is unlikely to care much about typography but a lot about the conditions of cancer, simply explained from his or her standpoint (and not merely as items of information from the physician's standpoint).[175]

Stephenson argues that simply bombarding people with facts or information does not work. Rather, individuals have to be approached in terms of what matters to them, which Stephenson boiled down to their values, beliefs, and opinions.[176] He says:

> Thus, in line with this theory, we do not give smokers information about the dangers of smoking, death rates, statistics or the like; *instead, we try to get them to cope with their smoking, as they understand it.*[177]

Stephenson further says this approach is not so simple as being "consumer-oriented" rather than "doctor-oriented." He considered it a matter of what people can *identify with.*

Stephenson also was critical of the typical health care film and pamphlet which tend to be fact-oriented. He urged the use of people-oriented material, developed from the standpoint of the consumer rather than the physician, educator, or communicator.[178]

Another important concept for Stephenson is that advertising and promotion—the act of informing people—does little good if the product or service promoted is unavailable. A *facilitator* often is necessary for action to take place. A facilitator can take the form of transportation for those who have no private way of reaching a doctor or hospital.[179] Stephenson thought effective communication also could be enhanced by a facilitator. This could be something as simple as a refrigerator magnet that listed phone numbers of health care providers or facilities.

Stephenson used Q methodology, which he described as a "highly quantitative" method, "making use of factor analysis and computer programming," to study values, beliefs, and opinions of both employees and patients of the Wayne Miner Neighborhood Heatlh Care Center.[180] He determined that people form images, or what he termed "schemata," of the world around them. It is possible to communicate to people only in terms of *their* schemata, Stephenson believed.[181]

Working in the 1960s, Stephenson found four schemata present in the population he studied. He described them as:

> One (A) was that of the relatively poor (lower middle class), which was in some sense fatalist and unhappy about medical matters in general, with no conceptions about how to deal with medical and health care problems at a national level. Another (B) was highly supportive of the medical profession as it was—of course physicians and nurses were so inclined. The third (C) was critical of medicine, feeling that something should be done for the aged and the poor. The fourth (D) were housewives who had a special relationship to physicians, chiefly through child care practices in the schools. No one, at that time (1965-67) displayed any feeling or belief in what would be describes as "socialized medicine" in other Western nations.[182]

Stephenson and his team of researchers used this information to develop a series of people-oriented pamphlets. His overall conclusion is that selecting content and design that are in accord with the various population schemata and then finding ways to facilitate the communication will result in the most effective communication possible.

CAMPAIGN EXAMPLES

Many health care campaigns have been planned, implemented, and evaluated. However, the Forsyth County Cervical Cancer Prevention Project, the Minnesota Heart Heatlh Care Program, the California Anti-Smoking Campaign, the Partnership for a Drug-Free American, Project Star, and the Stanford Five-City Heart Disease Prevention Project are summarized below because they represent projects that used both mass media and direct education approaches to attempt to change behaviors.

Forsyth County Cervical Cancer Prevention Project

Dignan et al. summarize the steps taken to establish a cervical cancer prevention project in Forsyth County, North Carolina. The project was designed to increasing the proportion of black women who obtain Pap smears on a regular basis and to encourage them to return for followup care when necessary. The ultimate goal was to reduce mortality.

The social marketing concept was selected as the model. Social marketing is based on the concept that marketing strategies can be used to influence the acceptability of social programs.[183]

The project utilized a combination of mass media and direct education to increasing participation in screening for cervical cancer in the target population. The project had two components designed to work together: 1) mass media to promote awareness and provide general information concerning cervical cancer and the important benefits of Pap smears, and 2) direct education (in small groups) to provide specific information to increase motivation and overcome barriers for high-risk, hard to reach women.[184]

The campaign developers expected to have to overcome through education the fear and fatalism at the mere mention of the word "cancer." Because they fear cancer, people can exhibit what the authors called the "psychologically protective, but medically dangerous, responses" such as the avoidance of physicians or the discounting of dissonant information (e.g., that some cancers can be cured if detected early). The authors also point out that the factors commonly associated with development of cervical cancer, early initiation of sexual intercourse and multiple partners, can be "perceived as negative, labeling statements."[185]

The role of focus groups within the social marketing model in this project concerned concept development to "flesh out" program objectives. The campaign planners began with focus groups to collect "information from the target population that would allow free expression of thoughts and feelings about cancer and related issues."[186] The planners used focus groups "to develop a conceptual framework for producing health care education materials addressing early detection of cervical cancer with the Pap smear."[187] They summarize the findings in this way:

All focus group participants reported that health care was among the most important elements of their lives. It is important to note, however, that for women with families this value did not apply as strongly to their own health care as to the health care of their family members—especially children. Personal health care was valued insofar as health care was necessary for the mother (or grandmother) to function appropriately. Prevention, accordingly, was said to be very important particularly in the context of family functioning.

Fear and fatalism were the primary reactions of the participants when cancer was discussed. In every group at least one individual related a story of a friend or relative who underwent treatment for cancer, suffered greatly and ultimately died. Cancer stories with positive outcomes were rare. When the moderator asked participants what their immediate reaction to a diagnosis of cancer would be, the responses were consistently fatalistic ("I would prepare to meet my maker." "I would begin arranging for someone to take care of my children.") Interestingly, the participants did not clearly differentiate cancer by type or site: In the midst of the focus group participants all cancer was the same, all cancer was fatal.

When asked if there was anything to be done to prevent cancer, the focus group participants concluded that prayer was the most important factor, followed by seeing a doctor promptly if there was any suspicion of disease. Delay in diagnosis was clearly identified as an important factor in the eventual outcome for cancer patients.[188]

The planners also note that there was a lack of knowledge about the Pap smear. They found unawareness of the relationship between the test and cervical cancer and misconceptions about the purpose of Pap smears, including beliefs that the Pap smear is a test for infection or pregnancy.[189]

Dignan et al. also discuss structural barriers that affect access, including policies of health care delivery systems, health providers' policies, transportation, child care, and long waiting times at doctors' offices for non-acute medical problems. They find competing financial obligations and transportation are most often mentioned by the focus group members as reasons why routine health care was not obtained. Also the justifications given for not consulting a physician when cancer is involved include: nothing can be done about the disease; the treatments are disfiguring, costly and ineffective; and, early diagnosis only produces a longer period of suffering.[190]

Dignan et al. say results from the focus groups provided the detail needed to apply the principles of social marketing to implementation of the program. Results influenced the production of public service announcements for radio and television, development of print mass media messages, and development of direct education for high risk women. Focus group results also guided the development of the overall theme for the project:

> Since the focus group participants agreed that seeing a doctor early could be important to the outcome with cancer, the theme, "early detection works" was selected as a simple, short, clear theme to illustrate the overall spirit and goal of the program. . . .

The fear and fatalism shown during the focus group discussion strongly suggested that a positive approach to early detection of cervical cancer would be more likely to be successful than an approach based on knowledge of the disease. Images and messages of the health education program were all designed to emphasize the value of early detection as a means of health enhancement rather than as a means of preventing cancer.[191]

Minnesota Heart Health Program

Another program that utilized mass media in combination with other elements is the Minnesota Heart Health Program. One of the major concerns of this project was how to bridge the knowledge gap. The theory behind the knowledge gap hypothesis was discussed previously. The main idea of this theory is:

> As the infusion of mass media information into a social system increases, segments of the population with higher socioeconomic status tend to acquire the information at a faster rate than the lower status segments, so that the gap between these segments tends to increase rather than decrease.[192]

Viswanath et al. say scholars have identified conditions under which knowledge gaps may or may not widen: 1) Gaps are less likely to widen when the topics are likely to appeal to lower socio-economic status (SES) groups. 2) Gaps are less likely when conflict is very high and the issue is of basic concern to the community. 3) Gaps are less likely when the community structure is homogeneous and when the sponsoring agencies are able to exercise greater degree of control over the environment. 4) Gaps are less likely to occur in the case of startling events which attract sustained media coverage.[193] On the other hand, gaps are more likely to occur when topics are more appealing to persons from higher SES than to lower SES respondents and when the topics are national in scope.[194]

For the Minnesota project, a variety of channels were used to deliver educational messages: 1) mass media; 2) direct education and adult education classes; 3) professional education by organizing workshops for physicians, dentists, nutritionists, nurses and other health professionals; 4) youth education; 5) environmental programs including grocery stores, restaurants, medical centers and work sites; and 6) community leaders and community organizations.[195] Mass media used included local radio, television, newspapers, videos, slide-tape programs, brochures, posters, and billboards.[196]

In addition, heart health centers recruited citizens to undergo screening for risk factors by contacting households in the target community. Risk factors included in the screenings were hypertension, cholesterol, physical activity level, and smoking. Participants were shown videotape presentations and counselled by the professional staff. Direct education courses, seminars and workshops also were available.

Part of the evaluation of this program included charting of knowledge gaps. Viswanath et al. report the following:

> In our analyses, we found that knowledge gaps did emerge and existed in some of our communities at different times. This was more often the case on knowledge about topics that have not been actively promoted in the campaigns. Most important, these minimal gaps in knowledge on campaign-emphasized knowledge were found in not only our two education communities but also in one of our reference communities. Only in the reference community did gaps close.[197]

They say gaps are found in "secular or non-emphasized knowledge, which was strongly associated with education in all communities." The gaps mostly occur with factors such as stress, caffeine consumption, and non-modifiable factors such as age, heredity and family history.

The authors conclude there are two policy implications that can be derived from the program evaluation:

First, knowledge gaps are not inevitable. Campaigns do lead to a wider distribution and often equalization of knowledge, when they are accompanied by other concomitants such as legitimization and redefinition of the issues by those in power. Once powerful groups in a social system identify a threat and take action to minimize the threat, the consequent dissemination of information on the factors and on the actions may lead to more equitable distribution of knowledge. This does not mean that there are no knowledge gaps. But the inequities are less pronounced and the definition of the issue must come from powerful groups in the system.

A second implication is that when some issues have not been definitely identified as a threat and are subject to a disagreement, or at least a lack of consensus among elites, knowledge gaps on that topic are more likely to emerge. One consequence of this is that the educated elite of a system enjoy more complete knowledge than the less education.[198]

In addition, the authors say that the more information moves out of the realm of specialized groups to the general public, the smaller the knowledge gap. They refer to this as a "supplementation" effect. Lazarsfeld and Merton suggest media effects are likely to be larger when information dissemination is accompanied by any of the three conditions: monopolization, canalization, and supplements. Consequently, gaps may not open or may close because of the "complementarity" of efforts by other organizations.[199]

Viswanath et al. say there are further implications for campaign planners. They conclude that "information campaigns in highly pluralistic communities may require higher commitment and that expectations of impact of campaigns in pluralistic systems even after five years have to be tempered."[200]

California Anti-Smoking Campaign

The Associated Press provides information about an anti-smoking campaign undertaken in California that led to a 28% drop in the number of smokers over five years, three times the national decline.[201] The California program is the result of a referendum called Proposition 99 passed in 1988 and financed by a 25-cent hike in the state cigarette tax. It includes school education programs, grants to cities and towns to develop workplace and restaurant smoking policies, and a series of advertisements such as one showing tobacco industry executives seated around a table in a smoke-filled room, chuckling and saying, "We're not in this business for our health."[202]

Teen-agers, the most receptive audience for cigarette advertisements, are the only group in which smoking did not decline, according to a five-year assessment report of the $599 million campaign. According to the Associated Press, the assessment also shows that bans on smoking in the workplace cut cigarette consumption by 26% and helped many smokers quit altogether. The ads and the grants to cities and towns are considered the most effective programs.

Interestingly, although about 37% of the tax money intended for the anti-smoking campaign was given to physicians, the evaluation found that advice from doctors did little to encourage quitting, and 51% of doctors didn't even tell smokers to quit. Furthermore, 25% of the budget funded school programs which were found to be ineffective, the report says.[203]

The Partnership for a Drug-Free America

Backer and Marson describe the Partnership for a Drug-Free America, founded in 1986, as a coalition of advertising agencies, television networks, publishers, trade associations, cable television companies, and other organizations, with the mission of using the power of advertising through the mass media to prevent drug abuse. In its first five years of operation, the Partnership placed more than $1 billion of pro bono public serve advertising in print, radio, and television media.[204]

The authors emphasize that the Partnership began its activities in 1986 "with a careful needs assessment and review of public-service advertising techniques, including dialogues with media campaign scholars and consults in academic positions." This assessment determined that the campaign should emphasize "the risks of drug use in order to capture attention and impress the national audience about the seriousness of the drug problem," from which the "fried egg" public service announcements ("This is your brain on drugs"). Other messages are aimed to make drug use look unglamorous and to build a climate of social intolerance for use.[205]

Although the authors offer no details of the planning process or evaluation, the follow-up messages included several targeted at minority communities. These messages were initially avoided to keep from contributing to a widespread misconception that drug use was only a problem among minorities.

Backer and Marson report that a national evaluation conducted by the Gordon S. Black Corporation indicated considerable awareness and attitude change among key target audiences such as American teenagers.[206] They say:

> "Unselling drugs" is complex. It involves many target groups, with very different types of messages needed to reach each (users, potential users, those who influence the behavior of users or potential users, etc.). In order to be effective, the "demoralization of drugs" campaign would consist of multiple messages delivered at many levels over a long period of time.[207]

Backer and Marson say major formative evaluation research was undertaken at the beginning of the antidrug campaign to determined more precisely which attitudes might be changed. The result was:

> The Partnership task force outlined advertising strategies based on available information, explained the drug adoption process, and recommended message ideas with which creative people should work in developing print and broadcast ads. Three drug abuse groups were targeted; eight target "markets" were identified (with several subgroups within these eight); several messages were outlined for each target and drug group; multiple media formats (print ads, radio ads, and television ads) were selected for each message; and numerous advertising agencies and creative talents were involved in developing the campaign.[208]

In addition to the media focus, messages also have been placed on posters; included in employee education programs; incorporated in schools and community prevention and treatment organization programs; and added to in-home video rentals and also used posters. Bracker and Marson credit the high quality of the advertising for the success of the program. They say national awareness surveys demonstrate that Partnership messages are among the best-recalled ads of all categories and that some, such as the fried egg commercial have been included into the American culture.[209]

Project Star

A substance program, the Midwestern Prevention Project (MPP), in Kansas City and Indianapolis describes the effects of community organization on a prevention campaign. Coincident with USC's preparation of a proposal (for community-based prevention research), in 1984, Ewing Kauffman, owner of the Kansas City Royals professional baseball team, chairman of the board of Marion Laboratories, and a noted philanthropist in Kansas City, sought assistance from the National Institute on Drug Abuse to initiate a citywide drug abuse prevention program for youth in Kansas City. Problems with drug abuse of several Kansas City Royals team members had stimulated his interest. In 1984, he asked USC for help in designing and evaluating a drug abuse prevention program that would capitalize on the recent mass media attention given to the Kansas City Royals' drug problem.[210]

The project used a proactive approach to drug abuse prevention with no initial mass media coverage in Indianapolis contrasted with an immediately reactive approach to drug abuse prevention with extensive mass media coverage in Kansas City. The authors describe the components below:

> The *mass media component* of the MPP consisted of approximately 31 television, radio, and print broadcasts per year about the rub abuse prevention intervention. . . .
>
> The *school program component* was delivered by trained teachers and included 10 to 13 classroom sessions in grades 6 or 7 (the transition year from elementary school to middle or junior high school), a 5-session booster in the following year, and peer counseling and support activities in high school. . . .
>
> The *parent program component* was delivered by a trained core group composed of the principal, four to six parents, and two student peer leaders from each school. The parent program included regular meetings throughout each school year to plan and implement an annual parent skills night for all parents, emphasizing parent-child communication and prevention support skills; to conduct monitoring activities to keep the school grounds and surrounding neighborhoods drug-free; and to refine school policy to institutionalize prevention programming in the school. . .
>
> The *community organization component* involved the identification, commitment, and training of existing city leaders to plan and implement drug abuse prevention services, to provide funds and other resources, and to carry out activities that complement other program components. . . .
>
> The *health policy change component* was implemented by a government subcommittee of the community organization leaders and other local government leaders. . . .[211]

A two-group research design is used to evaluate the effectiveness of the drug abuse prevention intervention. The drug-use and drug-use-related behaviors of adolescents in schools assigned to receive the program components directly is compared with adolescents in schools assigned to a "health-education-as-usual" control condition. The authors say the measurement design is "longitudinal, with samples of adolescents, their parents, school staff, adult community residents, and community leaders assessed annually through self-report surveys, telephone surveys, observation, archival records, and—for adolescents—a biochemical measure of cigarette smoking." Results indicate that while both groups of adolescents increase in drug use over time, adolescents in schools assigned to the intervention condition increase less and have consistently lower prevalence rates of cigarette, alcohol, and marijuana use than do adolescents in intervention school. They also show less cocaine and crack use compared to adolescents in control schools. Additionally, there has been a deceased alcohol and marijuana use among parents of adolescents in the intervention schools compared to the control schools and increased parent-child communication about drug-abuse prevention.[212]

The Stanford Five-City Heart Disease Prevention Project

The Stanford Five-City Project (FCP) is a long-term field trial designed to reduce cardiovascular disease (CVD) morbidity and mortality and risk. Flora et al. say the study employs a quasi-experimental design . . . with two treatment communities and three matched control communities. When the FCP was launched in 1978, it began with baseline data collection followed 1 1/2 years later by a six-year education program. The study is now in its 16th year with CVD monitoring still ongoing.[213] Among this program's major achievements are its successes with media and community organization involvement.

The authors say intervention effects were measured in the following manner:

A cohort of individuals aged 12 to 74 (were) surveyed approximately every 2 years for 8 years, and four cross-sectional samples (were) administered the same survey in years between the cohort surveys. After 5 1/3 years of the campaign, survey results show that relative to controls the cohort had a 16% decrease in coronary heart disease risk score and a 15% decrease in a composite total CVD mortality risk score. Decreased risk was produced by important changes in knowledge, blood pressure, smoking, and possibly blood cholesterol levels. The largest risk factor changes were achieved in blood pressure reductions and in smoking. Modest changes were achieved in weight control and diet.[214]

Mass media messages were transmitted in English and in Spanish via three television stations, three radio stations, three daily newspapers, and one weekly newspaper. Also, materials were mailed to people's homes and distributed in workplaces, grocery stores, pharmacies, physicians' offices, health agencies, hospitals, public libraries, and FCP offices.[215]

The specific components of the campaign include:

1. Television PSAs, news, and shows were a major component of the FCP campaign, with a total of 106 different television materials.
2. Radio was used primarily to reach the Spanish-speaking audience. . . .
3. Newspaper ads, columns, and feature stories resulted in the most unique newspaper messages. In newspapers, one of the most important FCP materials was the "Dr. Farquhar" column. (This column, published in English and Spanish newspapers, was designed to give up-to-date information on CVD, to interpret other information about CVD that was being disseminated via the media, to publicize local events about CVD risk reduction, to answer questions of readers, and to describe other CVD reduction efforts.)
4. Printed materials were distributed through the mail (tip sheets) or through mass distribution in workplace, physicians' offices, libraries, and healthcare agencies (booklets and brochures). These materials focused primarily on teaching community members skills they could use to change behavior.
5. Face-to-face presentations and curricula were used to supplement the mediated materials. These face-to-face programs took place in schools, workplace, social and fraternal organizations, and professional organizations (such as physicians' meeting in hospitals).[216]

The Project uses a communication behavior change framework, incorporating features of social cognitive theory, the theory of reasoned action, and the diffusion of innovations, to guide the development of the educational materials and campaign strategies. Social marketing, diffusion of innovations theory, and community adoption theory guided the dissemination and implementation of programs in the media and in schools, physicians' offices, health agencies, workplace, restaurants, grocery stores, and other organizations.[217]

The authors describe the main method used with organizations, community adoption theory in this way:

> The basic notion of community adoption theory is that little real development has occurred unless the community that is the target of change efforts feels a need for the change, participates in planning and executing the change program, takes some responsibility for the change program, and increasingly takes control of the change program. . . .[218]

Twelve guidelines were derived from community adoption theory and comprised the FCP community organization planning and implementation framework:

1. Identify community organizations and their perceptions of heart disease prevention, as well as their specific healthcare needs, perceptions, and domains of activity.
2. Study the interrelationships among the various groups and organizations in the community in order to understand and work through the existing power structure(s).
3. Utilize local community organizations to help develop and implement interventions.
4. Schedule interventions within the community context, for example, identify the appropriate times of the year when specific organizations are particularly eager to cooperate in project activities.
5. Tailor intervention programs according to the needs and perceptions on the part of individual consumers and organizations in the community.
6. Match the community organization's goals with those of the FCP.
7. Be alert to potential sources of conflict in the community regarding projectintervention and identify such barriers to cooperation before they become serious.
8. Provide linkages between project staff and community organizations so as to facilitate feedback and effective cooperation.

9. Create active involvement on the part of community organizations, so they will continue their efforts after the completion of the campaign.
10. Attempt to secure formal approval for long-range collaboration when obtaining organizational cooperation.
11. Provide inducement and incentives for both individual and organizational collaboration with the project.
12. Recognize community organizations as a process of problem solving, development, and action.[219]

Flora et al. conclude that mass media and other organizations are critical to the successful implementation of public communication campaigns:

> They serve as conduits of information, reinforce the change process, enhance resources applied to communication efforts, and insure the institutionalization of programs. Yet community organizations are often neglected participants in information campaigns. Studies of mass media campaigns typically discuss the project's theoretical underpinnings, interventions (messages), channels of communication, and effects of the campaign. Little attention is paid to the involvement of organizations, including the process of their recruitment, the nature of the involvement, and the outcomes of organizational participation.[220]

CONCLUSIONS

Perhaps one of the most important conclusion of this study is that there is a natural linkage among social marketing, network analysis, and Q methodology. None of the theories or examples reported above relied on Q methodology although much of what campaign planners need to accomplish can be determined through Q techniques. As the subsequent chapters will show, Q methodology can be used in the formative stages to determine community attitudes and to segment the audience within the innermost nest. Furthermore, Q techniques can help determine ranking ordering for the issues facing the community or target audience. Q methodology also can be linked to network analysis as discussed in Chapter III. Obviously, network analysis can be used to examine social groupings and diffusion patterns.

The following chapters will more thoroughly examine these links and demonstrate how Q methodology can be used in planning a health campaign that targets African Americans.

NOTES

1. William Stephenson, "The Vergent Report, April 1, 1967 - June 30, 1971" Western Historical Manuscript Collections, Ellis Library, University of Missouri, Columbia, I.

2. John S. Wright and Daniel S. Warner, *Advertising* (New York: McGraw-Hill Book Co., 1966), 408-409.

3. C.A. Kirkpatrick, *Advertising, Mass Communication in Marketing* (Boston: Houghton Mifflin Co., 1964), p. 345.

4. Brian R. Flay and Dee Burton, "Effective Mass Communication Strategies for Health Campaigns," in Charles Atkin and Lawrence Wallack, eds., *Mass Communication and Public Health: Complexities and Conflicts*, (Newbury Park, CA: Sage Publications, Inc., 1990), 130.

5. See E.M. Rogers and J.D. Storey, "Communication Campaigns," in C.R. Berger & S.H. Chaffee, eds., *Handbook of Communication Science*, (Newbury Park, CA: Sage Publications, Inc., 1988), 817-846; and Thomas E. Backer and Everett M. Rogers, eds., *Organizational Aspects of Health Communication Campaigns: What Works?*, (Newbury Park, CA: Sage Publications, Inc., 1993), 1-2.

6. Patricia G. Devine and Edward R. Hirt, "Message Strategies for Information Campaigns: A Social-Psychological Analysis," in Charles T. Salmon, ed., *Information Campaigns: Balancing Social Values and Social Change*, (Newbury Park, CA: Sage Publications, Inc., 1989), 230.

7. Brian R. Flay and Dee Burton, "Effective Mass Communication Strategies for Health Campaigns," in Charles Atkin and Lawrence Wallack, eds., *Mass Communication and Public Health: Complexities and Conflicts*, (Newbury Park, CA: Sage Publications, Inc., 1990), 131.

8. Ibid., 132.

9. Thomas E. Backer and Everett M. Rogers, eds., *Organizational Aspects of Health Communication Campaigns: What Works?*, (Newbury Park, CA: Sage Publications, Inc., 1993), 2.

10. Robert Abbot Olins, "A Model Study of an Advertising Campaign" (Ph.D. diss., University of Missouri, 1971), 6.

11. Donald F. Cox, "Clues for Advertising Strategists II," *Harvard Business Review*, 39(6), (1961): 162.

12. Olins, 11-12.

13. G.D. Wiebe, "Merchandising Commodities and Citizenship on Television," *Public Opinion Quarterly*, XXV (1951), 679.

14. Charles T. Salmon, "Campaigns for Social 'Improvement': An Overview of Values, Rationales, and Impacts," in Charles T. Salmon, ed., *Information Campaigns: Balancing Social Values and Social Change*, (Newbury Park, CA: Sage Publications, Inc., 1989), 21-24.

15. Ibid., 25.

16. Lawrence M. Wallack, "Mass Media Campaigns: The Odds Against Finding Behavior Change," *Health Education Quarterly* 8(3), (Fall, 1981): 210.

17. Ibid., 220.

18. Ibid.

19. Ibid., 443.

20. Wallack, 222.

21. J.F. Mosher and L.M. Wallack, "Proposed Reforms in the Regulation of Alcoholic Beverage Advertising," *Contemporary Drug Problem*, 8 (1979), 87-106 quoted in Wallack, 234.

22. M.P. Stern et al., "Results of a Two-Year Health Education Campaign on Dietary Behavior," *Circulation*, 54, (1976) 826-833, cited in Wallack, 220.

23. R.T. LaPiere, "Attitude vs. Action," *Social Forces*, 13 (1934): 230-237.

24. I. Deutscher, "Words and Deeds: Social Science and Social Policy, " reprinted from *Social Problems*, 13 (1966) 233-254, in *The Sociologist as Detective*, ed. W. Saunders, (New York: Praeger Publishers, 1976), 39.

25. A.W. Wicker, "Attitudes Versus Actions: The Relationship of Verbal and Overt Behavioral Responses to Attitude Objects," *Journal of Social Issues*, 45 (1969), 65 .

26. Wallack, 238.

27. I. Ajzen and M. Fishbein, "Attitude-Behavior Relations: A Theoretical Analysis and Review of Empirical Research," *Psychological Bulletin*, 84, (1977), 888-918.

28. Wallack, 238.

29. S.J. Gross and C. Niman, "Attitude Behavior Consistency: A Review," *Public Opinion Quarterly*, 39, (1975), 912 .

30. Ibid.

31. Wallack, 240.

32. Ibid., 241.

33. Richard K. Manoff, *Social Marketing: New Imperative for Public Health*, (New York: Praeger Publishers, 1985), 53.

34. See G.D. Wiebe, "Merchandising Commodities and Citizenship on Television," *Public Opinion Quarterly*, 15, 679-691; and Charles T. Salmon, ed., *Information Campaigns: Balancing Social Values and Social Change*, (Newbury Park, CA: Sage Publications, Inc.), 19.

35. Manoff, 3-4.

36. Ibid., 4.

37. Charles Atkin and Lawrence Wallack, eds., *Mass Communication and Public Health: Complexities and Conflicts*, (Newbury Park, CA: Sage Publications, Inc., 1990), 155.

38. Ibid.

39. Ibid., 156.

40. Ibid., 157.

41. Charles T. Salmon, "Campaigns for Social 'Improvement': An Overview of Values, Rationales, and Impacts," in Charles T. Salmon, ed., *Information Campaigns: Balancing Social Values and Social Change*, (Newbury Park, CA: Sage Publications, Inc., 1989), 21.

42. Manoff, 16.

43. Ibid.

44. Ibid., 17.

45. Ibid.

46. Ibid.

47. Ibid., 18.

48. Robert Hornik, "The Knowledge-Behavior Gap in Public Information Campaigns: A Development Communication View,"in Charles T. Salmon, ed., *Information Campaigns: Balancing Social Values and Social Change*, (Newbury Park, CA: Sage Publications, Inc., 1989), 114.

49. Ibid., 121.

50. Ibid., 122.

51. Ibid., 125.

52. Ibid., 128.

53. Ibid.

54. Ibid., 35.

55. Ibid., 42.

56. Ibid., 103.

57. Ibid., 99.

58. Flay and Burton, 157.

59. Hertog, 2.

60. Ibid., 2-3.

61. Ibid., 5.

62. Ibid.

63. Ibid.

64. Ibid.

65. Ibid.

66. Ibid.

67. William J. Brown, "Effects of an AIDS Prevention Campaign on Attitudes, Beliefs, and Communication Behavior," Paper presented at the Health

Communication Division of the 41st Annual Conference of the International Communication Association, Chicago, 25 May 1991, 5.

68. Ibid.

69. Ibid.

70. Flay and Burton, 157.

71. Ibid., 158.

72. Leon Quera, *Advertising Campaigns: Formulation and Tactics*, 2d ed., (Columbus, Ohio: Grid Inc., 1977), 1.

73. Ibid.

74. Ibid.

75. Ibid., 2.

76. Ibid., 10.

77. Ibid., 17.

78. Ibid.

79. Ibid., 25.

80. Ibid., 67.

81. Ibid., 129.

82. Ibid.

83. Ibid., 187.

84. Ibid., 188.

85. J. Fitzpatrick, *Puerto Rican Americans: The Meaning of Migration to the Mainland*, (Englewood Cliffs, N.J.: Prentice-Hall, 1971) quoted in Vicente Abad, Juan Ramos and Elizabeth Boyce, "A Model for Delivery of Mental Health Services to Spanish-Speaking Minorities," *American Journal of Orthopsychiatry*, 44 (4), (July 1974), 590.

86. F. Reissman et al., eds., *Mental Health of the Poor*, (New York: The Free Press, 1964) quoted in Abad, Ramos and Boyce, 591.

87. James Hertog et al., "Formative Analysis for Community-Based Health Campaigns: Experiences of the Cancer and Dietary Intervention Project," Paper presented at the Health Communication Division of the 41st Annual Conference of the International Communication Association, Chicago, 25 May 1991, 6.

88. Ibid.

89. Ibid., 7.

90. Ibid., 11.

91. Charles K. Atkin, Gina M. Garramone and Ronald Anderson, "Formative Evaluation Research in Health Campaign Planning: The Case of Drunk Driving Prevention," Paper presented at annual conference of International Communication Association, Health Communication Division, Chicago, May 1986, 3.

92. Ibid.

93. Ibid, 3-4.

94. Ibid., 5.

95. Ibid.

96. Ibid.

97. Ibid., 5-6.

98. Ibid., 6.

99. Ibid.

100. Ibid., 7.

101. Everett M. Rogers and F. Floyd Shoemaker, *Communication of Innovations*, (New York: The Free Press, 1971), 244-245.

102. Arun Sharma, "The Persuasive Effect of Salesperson Credibility: Conceptual and Empirical Examination," *Journal of Personal Selling & Sales Managements*, 10 (Fall 1990), 71.

103. Ibid., 72.

104. Ibid.

105. Ibid.

106. Ibid., 73.

107. Ibid.

108. Ibid., 8.

109. Manoff, 48.

110. James E. Grunig, "Publics, Audiences and Market Segments: Segmentation Principles for Campaigns," in Charles T. Salmon, ed., *Information Campaigns: Balancing Social Values and Social Change*, (Newbury Park, CA: Sage Publications, Inc., 1989), 199.

111. Ibid., 202-203.

112. Ibid., 203.

113. Ibid., 204.

114. Ibid.

115. Ibid., 206.

116. Ibid.

117. Ibid., 206, 219.

118. Ibid., 209.

119. See H. Assael, *Consumer Behavior and Marketing Action*, 2d. ed., (Boston: Kent Publishers, 1984), 167, and Grunig, 209.

120. Grunig, 210.

121. Ibid., 211.

122. Ibid., 211.

123. Ibid., 213.

124. Ibid., 216-217.

125. Ibid., 219-220.

126. Ibid., 221.

127. Ibid., 219.

128. Ibid., 218.

129. Hornik, 126.

130. Grunig, 221.

131. Ibid., 222.

132. Ibid.

133. Atkin, Garramone, and Anderson, 8.

134. Gerald J.S. Wilde, "Effects of Mass Media Communications on Health and Safety Habits: An Overview of Issues and Evidence," *Addiction* 88 (1993): 986-987.

135. Flay and Burton, 135-136.

136. Ibid., 136.

137. Ibid., 133-134.

138. Devine and Hirt., 243-244.

139. Grunig, 251-252.

140. Charles Atkin and Elaine Bratic Arkin, "Issues and Initiatives in Communicating Health Information to the Public, " in Charles Atkin and Lawrence Wallack, eds., *Mass Communication and Public Health: Complexities and Conflicts*, (Newbury Park, CA: Sage Publications, Inc., 1990), 13.

141. Ibid., 14.

142. Ibid., 20.

143. Manoff, 75-76.

144. Ibid., 76-77.

145. P. Shoemaker, "Deviance of Political Groups and Media Treatment," *Journalism Quarterly* 61 (1984): 66-75.

146. Philip Meyer, "News Media Responsiveness to Public Health," in Charles Atkin and Lawrence Wallack, eds., *Mass Communication and Public Health: Complexities and Conflicts*, (Newbury Park, CA: Sage Publications, Inc., 1990), 53.

147. John R. Finnegan, Jr., Neil Bracht, and K. Viswanath, "Community Power and Leadership Analysis in Lifestyle Campaigns," in Charles T. Salmon, ed., *Information Campaigns: Balancing Social Values and Social Change*, (Newbury Park, CA: Sage Publications, Inc., 1989), 55.

148. Ibid., 54.

149. Ibid., 55.

150. Ibid., 56-57.

151. Ibid.

152. Ibid.

153. Ibid., 58.

154. Salmon, 40-41.

155. Devine and Hirt, 230-231.

156. Ibid., 232-233.

157. Grunig, 251.

158. Ibid., 252-253.

159. Manoff, 49-50.

160. Ibid., 68-69.

161. Ibid., 69.

162. Atkin and Arkin, 34-35.

163. Ibid., 35.

164. Ibid.

165. Ibid., 36.

166. Ibid., 141.

167. Ibid., 144.

168. Ibid., 145-146.

169. Eric Adler, "A Race at Risk," *The Kansas City Star*, 24 July 1991, A8.

170. Ibid.

171. Ibid.

172. Ibid.

173. Ibid.

174. Ibid.

175. Stephenson, i.

176. Ibid., 3.

177. Ibid., 4.

178. Ibid., 4-5.

179. Ibid., 5.

180. Ibid., 7.

181. Ibid., 9.

182. Ibid., 14.

183. R.C. Lefebvre and J.A. Flora, "Social Marketing and Public Health Interventions," *Health Education Quarterly*, 15, (1988), 299-315, cited in Mark Dignan, "The Role of Focus Groups in Health Education for Cervical Cancer Among Minority Women," *Journal of Community Health*, 15 (6), (December 1990): 374.

184. Mark Dignan, "The Role of Focus Groups in Health Education for Cervical Cancer Among Minority Women," *Journal of Community Health*, 15 (6), (December 1990): 374.

185. Ibid., 370.

186. Ibid.

187. Ibid., 370-371.

188. Ibid., 372.

189. Ibid., 373.

190. Ibid., 374.

191. Ibid., 374-375.

192. P.J. Tichenor, G.A. Donohue, and C.N. Olien, *Community Conflict and the Press*, (Beverly Hills, CA: Sage, 1980), 159-160.

193. K. Viswanath et al., "Health and Knowledge Gaps: Some Lessons from the Minnesota Heart Health Program," Paper presented to the annual conference of the International Communication Association, Chicago, IL, 23-27 May 1991, 3.

194. Ibid.

195. Ibid., 6.

196. Ibid.

197. Ibid., 7.

198. Ibid., 8-9.

199. Ibid., 9-10.

200. Ibid., 12.

201. The Associated Press, "Report Attests to Success of Calif. Anti-Smoking Campaign," *The Daily Advocate*, 21 March 1994, 12A.

202. Ibid.

203. Ibid.

204. Thomas E. Backer and Ginna Marston, "Partnership for a Drug-Free America: An Experiment in Social Marketing," in Thomas E. Backer and Everett M. Rogers, eds., *Organizational Aspects of Health Communication Campaigns: What Works?*, (Newbury Park, CA: Sage Publications, Inc., 1993), 10.

205. Ibid., 11.

206. Ibid.

207. Ibid., 13-14.

208. Ibid., 14.

209. Ibid., 19.

210. Mary Ann Pentz and Thomas W. Valente, "Project Star: A Substance Abuse Prevention Campaign in Kansas City," in Thomas E. Backer and Everett M. Rogers, eds., *Organizational Aspects of Health Communication Campaigns: What Works?*, (Newbury Park, CA: Sage Publications, Inc., 1993), 39.

211. Ibid., 41-42.

212. Ibid., 43-44.

213. June A. Flora et al., "The Stanford Five-City Heart Disease Prevention Project," in Thomas E. Backer and Everett M. Rogers, eds., *Organizational Aspects of Health Communication Campaigns: What Works?*, (Newbury Park, CA: Sage Publications, Inc., 1993), 102-103.

214. Ibid., 103.

215. Ibid., 104.

216. Ibid., 105.

217. Ibid., 105-106.

218. Ibid., 106.

219. Ibid., 106-107.

220. Ibid., 101-102.

CHAPTER V

African American Media Habits

Remarkably, there appears to be little consistent effort to examine African Americans as a defined group of consumers. There are likely several reasons for this. First, a large segment of the African American market is not viewed as affluent consumers who will buy large quantities of luxury items. Second, and perhaps more importantly, mass media advertising is assumed to be as effective for black consumers as for white consumers. Until the 1980s, African Americans were never featured in television ads except in images of servitude (the Aunt Jemima syndrome). Today, the most prominent ads featuring black actors are selling KFC chicken and Phillips Milk of Magnesia, hardly an improvement in fighting stereotypes. There are some exceptions, such as black models selling cosmetics and various athletes or entertainers selling fast food, athletic shoes, or soft drinks to African Americans, but by and large commercials feature white faces. It has been left to the black newspapers and especially black magazines to build ads specifically designed for an African American audience. Billboards also have been used in inner city areas to sell products, chiefly tobacco and alcohol products. Consequently, there are few studies that specifically deal with an African American mass media audience.

THE BLOCK STUDY

In 1970 Carl Block, a business and public administration professor at the University of Missouri-Columbia, supervised face-to-face interviews with 350 residents (both black and white) in inner-city St. Louis.[1] Even though those interviewed had household incomes of $4,000 or less in 1970 dollars,

Block found that ownership of radio and television sets was about 84%. Slightly more than 70% claimed they were regular television viewers while 58% said they regularly listened to the radio. Radio was viewed as a source of music first and as a means of keeping informed on news, weather and sports second. In terms of television viewing, soap operas were the most popular shows, followed by news, weather and sports; adventure programs; and comedy programs.[2]

Block found that although the print media's reach was less than that of radio and television, nearly two-thirds of those interviewed at least looked at a newspaper almost every day. Additionally, 40% claimed to read at least one magazine every week.[3]

He concluded that based on the study's results:

> . . . television and newspapers are the two most effective modes of communication for reaching the urban poor. Both of these forms of mass media have high rates of exposure and involvement among those interviewed. . . .
>
> Newspapers and television were also listed as the two most useful sources in helping these individuals choose a product, that is, help them to get the most for their money.[4]

Block noted that 40% of those interviewed said they either did not read at all or read less than one hour per week. He said this means that "these people are almost completely cut off from a wealth of information that could be very valuable to them personally."[5]

Block also noted that there were only a few differences in attitudes between blacks and whites in his study. He found a significant relationship between race and the sources of information a person feels will be most helpful to him/her in choosing a product. The white respondents favored impersonal sources (media) rather than personal contact (family, friends, sales clerks, etc.). Although both groups placed newspapers and television at the top of their lists in terms of helpful sources, 41% of the white subjects, compared to 26% of the black subjects listed newspapers as their first choice. Almost 17% of the white subjects mentioned television, compared to 24% of the black subjects. Advice from friends was ranked third among the black respondents, but was ranked sixth among the white respondents. He said that 24% of the black subjects mentioned personal sources in general as the most useful in providing product information, compared to about 15% of the white subjects.[6]

Block found that 16% of the black subjects said they read a black-oriented magazine (*Ebony* was mentioned by 13%). He said a similar pattern exists for black radio. Also, 58% of the black subjects reacted favorably toward radio and television commercials in general, compared to 27% of the white subjects.[7]

Block also emphasizes the importance of formal education. He points out that the best educated earn more money, are more perceptive in their role as consumers, and generally lead a more comfortable life. Also, the higher the education level, the higher the amount of reading that takes place.[8] He found another interesting phenomenon:

> When little reading is done the greatest emphasis is placed upon convenience store locations as a factor in selecting a food outlet while less importance is placed on price. Those who read the most (i.e., the group which read at least three hours per week) placed greatest importance upon food prices and less on store location. . . .[9]

Block suggests two reasons for this: 1) those who spend the most time reading are better educated and, therefore, more perceptive generally; and 2) as individuals read more they generally increase their chances of being exposed to specific information concerning meal preparation and food purchasing. Block also found that men spent more time reading than did women.[10]

Block offers this concluding comment:

> The results of this study show that the mass media do reach the urban poor. This should provide sufficient evidence to encourage greater interest in the use of the mass media as a means of channeling much needed information to the poor on a number of subjects which directly affect their well-being.[11]

The question then, is how much has changed in the decades since Block investigated the habits of the urban poor in St. Louis? Could his observation about the correlation between reading and convenience store shopping today apply to the use of the emergency room for "convenient" health care? Has the proliferation of the computer and cable television even further reduced reading or created an even bigger gap between the urban poor and the affluent suburbanites?

AMALGAMATED PUBLISHER, INC., BLACK NEWSPAPER READERSHIP

Two more recent studies look at the readers of black newspapers across the country. A black newspaper refers to a newspaper that is published primarily for an African American audience and is often circulated in areas where African American households are concentrated.

The first of the two surveys was conducted in 1987 by Scarborough for Amalgamated Publishers, Inc. (API), the national advertising representative for 83 leading black community newspapers, including the Kansas City Call, the St. Louis Argus, the St. Louis Sentinel, and the St. Louis American.

The report indicates that the black consumer market has risen from about $100 billion when Block was conducting his survey in 1970 to $240 billion in 1990. Much of this growth has occurred since 1985.[12]

Among other things, this study found that about 47% of API readers consumed an alcoholic beverage in the month prior to the survey. Almost 35% smoke cigarettes.[13] The following table[14], using rounded Scarborough Research Corp. statistics and more recent figures prepared by TMN Research, Inc. For API, compares newspaper reader demographics to those of the general black population.

SEARS FOUNDATION/NNPA BLACK NEWSPAPER STUDY

The second study of relevance here is the Sears Foundation/National Newspaper Publishers Association study[15] of black newspaper readers conducted by the University of Missouri Media Research Bureau (under the direction of the author) in 1993. A total of 2,522 African American households in the Los Angeles, Ca.; Columbus, Ohio; Philadelphia, Pa.; Pittsburgh, Pa.; Houston, Texas; Winston-Salem, N.C.; and Birmingham, Al., areas were contacted by telephone.

TABLE 1
COMPARISON OF API READERS TO THE
AFRICAN AMERICAN POPULATION

	Black Population	1987 API Readers	1997 API Readers
N=	11,006,000	1,869	
Gender			
Male	44%	45%	53%
Female	56%	55%	47%
Age			
18-24	22%	14%	——
25-34	27%	23%	——
35-54	29%	36%	——
55+	23%	27%	53%
Education			
Post Graduate	3%	4%	43%
College Grad.	12%	14%	66%
Some College	20%	23%	——
High School Grad.	40%	37%	——
Not H.S. Grad.	25%	22%	——
Household Income			
30,000+	37%	30%	60%*
15,000-29,999	35%	36%	——
10,000 or less	28%	34%	——
*Estimated from figures provided.			
Occupation			
White collar	33%	38%	58%
Professional	16%	19%	——
Clerical/sales	17%	20%	——
Blue collar 13%	12%	——	
Marital Status			
Married	42%	48%	53%
Never married	35%	25%	22%
Separated/			
widowed/divorced	23%	27%	25%

TABLE 1 *(continued)*

	Black Population	1987 API Readers	1997 API Readers
Household Size			
5 or more	26%	23%	——
3 or 4	36%	37%	——
2	24%	27%	——
1	14%	13%	——
Number of Children			
One or more	54%	53%	——
One	19%	25%	——
Two+	35%	28%	——
Three+	15%	14%	——
Home Ownership			
Own home	47%	49%	85%
Condominium	.4%	.5%	——
Private home	46%	48%	——
Other	6%	3%	——
Electronic Equipment			
Color TV	83%	91%	——
Large Screen TV	22%	22%	——
VCR	37%	39%	——
Compact disc	9%	14%	——
Stereo/hi-fi	62%	68%	——
Personal Computer	13%	16%	——

Eighty-two percent of those contacted said there is a black newspaper serving their community. Sixty-eight percent personally read a black newspaper. Of those reading a black newspaper, 89% spend 15 minutes or more reading each issue. In addition, 44% said at least one other person in the household reads a black newspaper, with 75% saying two or more persons in the household read one. The major reason for reading a black newspaper is to get information that does not appear in the mainstream press, specifically information about the local community. Additionally, 74% either subscribe to or read a white or mainstream newspaper.

Eighty-two percent indicated they are likely to read health information if it clearly deals with special health problems blacks face. Also, 67% indicated they regularly and 27% indicated they occasionally read health information in their black newspapers. Fifty-six percent said they read articles about health in mainstream newspapers or magazines regularly, while 31% read them occasionally. Those who said they regularly or occasionally read health articles (2,154 respondents) were asked to provide the one type of health article they are most likely to read. They said:

General health	17%
AIDS	17%
Heart disease/high blood pressure	14%
Cancer	10%
Diet/nutrition	9%
Exercise	5%
Diabetes	5%
Diseases of the elderly	3%
Child/infant health	2%
Sickle Cell Anemia	2%
Stress	1%
Glaucoma/eye disease	1%

Fifty-two percent said they generally believe the articles on health they read, while 39% usually question their accuracy, and 9% said their belief depends on the source or the subject.

Sixty-seven percent of those interviewed said within the past two years they have made some change in their lifestyles, such as to quit smoking or to change the way they eat or the amount they exercise, to improve their own or their family's health.

Seventy-five percent buy or read at least one black magazine every month. Most read three or more. *Ebony* is the most popular, followed by *Jet* and *Essence*.

Seventy-five percent said they listen to a black radio station Monday through Friday. The average respondent listens 7.8 hours a week. In addition, 58% listen to a black radio station on weekends. The average number of listening hours is 5.1. The majority said they listen to the radio primarily for music or a combination of music and news. Thirty-two percent said they had patronized a store or business because of ads they had heard on the radio during the previous month.

Ninety-six percent said they watch or listen to television regularly. The average number of hours spent is 20.5. Entertainment shows are the favorite content (35%), followed by news (26%), and sports (11%). The least favorite types of shows are soap operas (8%) and game shows (7%). Additionally, 63% have cable television or a satellite dish. (This varied from as low as 50% in Houston to as high as 76% in Winston Salem.) Seventy-five percent have a VCR, and nearly 69% said they regularly or occasionally fast forward through commercials when they are watching pre-recorded programs. Thirty-eight percent said they had patronized a store or business in the previous month because of advertising they saw on television.

Twelve percent said they had patronized a store or business in the previous month because of a billboard advertisement, and 45% said they had patronized a store or business in the previous month because of a circular received in the mail. About 44% said they shop by mail at least occasionally.

The average amount of money spend on alcoholic beverages in a month is about $23, while about $22 are spent on cigarettes.

One of the rather surprising results of this study is that when the respondents were asked if they pay more attention to general advertising or to advertising that is specifically designed to appeal to minority groups, only 16% said minority advertising appeals to them more. Fifty-two percent said general advertising appeals to them more, while 13% said both appeal to them equally, and 19% said they never pay attention to advertising at all. The subjects were asked why they responded as they did. Most of those who prefer minority advertising do so because they want to support black businesses or they like feeling singled out for special consideration. However, the vast majority said they were simply interested in product or business attributes or objected to being "segregated" through advertising. Some interpreted a preference for black advertising as a form of racism. The following table shows the comparison between the Scarborough data and the Sears Foundation projects:

TABLE 2
SEARS FOUNDATION/NNPA READERS COMPARED TO
THE AFRICAN AMERICAN POPULATION

	Black Population	Sears/NNPA Readers
N=	11,006,000	2,522
Gender		
Male	44%	46%
Female	56%	54%
Age		
18-24	22%	Mean Age 43.8
25-34	27%	
35-54	29%	
55+	23%	
Education		
Post Graduate	3%	9%
College Grad.	12%	20%
Some College	20%	31%
High School Grad.	40%	31%
Not High School Grad.	—	10%
Household Income		
30,000+	37%	50%
15,000-29,999	35%	25%
10,000 or less	28%	7%
Occupation		
White collar	33%	47%
Professional	16%	28%
Clerical/sales	17%	19%
Blue collar 13%	45%	
Marital Status		
Married	42%	37%
Never married	35%	36%
Separated/ widowed/divorced	23%	28%
Number of Children		
One or more	54%	42%
One	19%	20%
Two+	35%	22%
Three+	15%	10%

These studies provide some understanding of the difficulties in reaching African American audiences. Although specialized media, such as black newspapers and radio stations, obviously do attract a large percentage of the target audience, such media does not always exist, and even if they do, they cannot always be persuaded to assist with a campaign, especially a health campaign. Part of the difficulty is that tobacco and alcohol companies pump large sums of money into these media. (The 1993 National Newspaper Publishers Association convention was sponsored by Anheuser Bush and Coors, for example.) In many cases, the newspaper or radio station would not survive without such support. It is editorially difficult, then, for these media to suggest that such products are literally killing their readers or listeners.

NOTES

1.   Carl E. Block, "Communicating with the Urban Poor: an Exploratory Inquiry," *Journalism Quarterly*, (Spring, 1970), 4.

2. Ibid., 5-6.

3. Ibid., 6.

4. Ibid.

5. Ibid.

6. Ibid., 7.

7. Ibid., 10.

8. Ibid., 8.

9. Ibid., 9.

10. Ibid.

11. Ibid., 11.

12. *Scarborough Report on Black Newspaper Audience Readership*, (New York: Amalgamated Publishers, Inc., 1987), 4.

13. Ibid., 21-22.

14. Ibid., 7-15, 23.

15. Judith Sylvester, Media Research Bureau Black Newspaper Readership Report, 24 June 1993, 1-48.

CHAPTER VI

Using Q Methodology to Determine Attitudes Toward the American Health System: An African American Perspective

Because African Americans face a myriad of health problems, many of which are preventable or manageable with medical treatment and because the reasons for the discrepancies between the general health state of African Americans compared to the white population are not clear, a new research approach is needed. Low socioeconomic status is most often cited as the major reason for the discrepancies, but this rationale does not explain why similar problems are less likely to be manifested in poor white and Hispanic populations or why African Americans at all income levels are generally in poorer health than the rest of the population. This puzzle has lead to new research using Q methodology, focus groups and survey research to examine segments of African American *attitudes* toward the health care system.

Q methodology, which was developed by William Stephenson, a former professor of journalism at the University of Missouri, is concerned with the way people react to statements of opinion. He believed the fundamental difference between objectivity and subjectivity is a matter of "self-reference:"

> . . . modern science has prospered by eliminating whims and arbitrary subjectivities from its fact-finding missions into the world "outside." Q methodology follows the same prescriptions for what we consider "inside"

us, matters of mind, consciousness, wishes and emotions, and it does so in terms of theories, universals, and laws, precisely as for modern physics.[1]

Patterson, who worked with Stephenson and used this methodology in her dissertation in 1966, summarized Stephenson's ideas:

> Given a large number of statements of opinion about a complex of communication, a sample can be taken for study. . .either a random selection from the large number, or a "representative" sample to fit a balanced block designed for the main effects which apparently are at issue.[2]

For a more thorough explanation of Q methodology, see Appendix A.

Although focus group interviews, used since the 1930s, are useful for instrument development, illustration, sensitization, or conceptualization,[3] for this research they were used to gain a better understanding of African American health concerns, to test terminology, formulate hypotheses and especially to elicit statements for the Q sort.

The first group for this study was convened in St. Louis, Mo., on Aug. 25, 1992, with members of a diabetes support group that meets at St. Louis County Hospital in the inner city area. Because more than 30 people were in attendance and no control was exercised over those who attended, it was more of a group discussion than a traditional focus group. The second group, held Jan. 25, 1993, consisted of people who were involved in several screening clinics sponsored by the Black Health Care Coalition in Kansas City, Mo. The participants were selected by the Coalition director. The other two groups, held Jan. 9, 1993, in St. Louis, Mo., and March 27, 1993, in Atlanta, Ga., were part of the Sears Foundation/National Newspaper Publishers Association project designed to help redesign African American newspapers. A health page was included in the discussion at both groups. Participants for the first group were selected from volunteers who responded to a newspaper ad and provided their ages. Participants in the Atlanta group were selected by several black newspaper publishers. Although the selection process was somewhat haphazard, participants did have varied demographic and socioeconomic background. Some worked in the health care field, some had regular contact with physicians as patients, and some had little personal contact with the health care system.

Additional Q sort statements were collected from presentations and papers given during the 4th Biennial Symposium on Minorities, the Medically Underserved & Cancer: Cultural Diversity, Poverty, and Health Care Reform April 21-24, 1993, in Houston, Texas. Presenters included primary care physicians, medical researchers, cancer survivors, and representatives of various health care support organizations.

For this study, the following underlying structures were selected:

1. Specific problems of blacks (7 statements)
2. Facilitators (3 statements)
3. Attitudes toward the health care system (7 statements)
4. Attitudes toward health (9 statements)
5. Access (14 statements)
6. Prevention (2 statements)
7. Health information (7 statements)

These 49 statements of opinion, selected from more than 200 self-referent statements collected, composed the Q sample. The selected statements best represent all the statements collected, and they fit into the underlying structures established to determine attitudes about health in general, about the health care system and providers, and about sources of information. The hope was that these statements would determine which subjects are concerned about access, barriers to health care, racism, etc., and then determine which health care campaign methods or modes of distribution will be most effective.

A list of people who had participated in the St. Louis focus groups and the Texas conference was the starting point for selecting subjects for this study. Approximately 100 people were selected based on their known demographics (age and race in particular). These people were sent the Q sort statements and instructions by mail. Additional people living in Missouri and Louisiana were selected through personal invitation, an advertisement in a church newsletter, and through contacts in the Louisiana State University maintenance department. These subjects were either sent the questionnaire through the mail or were given to them by their work supervisor. Every effort was made to get a balance of males and females, blacks and whites, and high and low income and education levels. In addition, several physicians were asked to participate. In all about 135 people were asked to do the sorts, and all but the LSU employees who participated were paid $10 if they returned the completed materials. Because some subjects were never reached because of outdated addresses and some refused to participate, a total of 57 Q sorts were collected.

Although Q methodology is effective in determining attitude clusters, it has been criticized as being limited because results cannot be projected to the great population the way sampling research often can. To overcome this weakness, an additional step was undertaken. A telephone survey of 527 adults from St. Louis, Kansas City, and Baton Rouge, La., was conducted to determine what percentage of the greater population might fall into the defined factors. The results of this survey will be discussed in Chapter VIII and Chapter IX.

FACTOR ANALYSIS

Factor analysis is a statistical procedure that treats all variables as equals. Weiers offers the following advantages of factor analysis:

> In marketing research studies, we may end up with a large number of measurements, or variables for a set of respondents. This can lead to two difficulties: (1) the sheer number of variables may be a bit unwieldy for further analysis; and (2) some of the variables may be highly related to others, leading to reliability problems such as multicollinearity Factor analysis can help reduce the number of variables to a level that is easier to manage, but that still contains most of the information found in the (much larger) original set.[4]

He further states that this method starts with a "matrix of correlations between variables" and proceeds to generate "new" variables (factors), "each of which is a linear combination of the original variable."[5]

It is important to note that Q methodology involves a major difference from traditional factor analysis in the way factors are defined. Rather than factoring the statements in the Q sort, the subjects (people) themselves form the factors. Thus, when factors are mentioned in this study, it is groups of people who are being described.

RESULTS

The factor analysis of 57 subjects yielded five types worthy of interpretation. (One person did not correlate with any factor, so the analysis is actually based on 56 responses.) For purposes of analysis, these groups will be called (1) The Equalizers (2) The Preventers (3) The Empathizers, (4) The Adjusters and (5) The Fixers. These types are described in detail in Chapter VII.

FACTOR ROTATION

PCQuanl uses varimax rotation, which "attempts to 'clean up' the factors in the factor loading table, that is, force the entries in the columns to be near 0 or 1."[6] For this study, principal component factoring produced five types with eigenvalues greater than 1.00. Brown points out that "the significance of a factor is somehow related to its 'strength' as measured by the magnitude of its eigenvalue or, equivalently, in terms of the percentage of total variance accounted for." He said that relying on an eigenvalue greater than 1.00 is widespread but quite arbitrary. For example, Brown said in a study he conducted only one person loaded significantly on a factor. However, that person was a decision-maker whose attitudes and opinions were of great value to the study.[7] Similarly for this study, although a four-factor solution was considered, the subjects who indicated they believe illness can be a punishment from God are best isolated by a five-factor solution. Additionally, the five-factor solution produced a predominately white type, two predominately black types and two other types that, although racially mixed, showed differing economic and educational backgrounds. Thus, the five-factor solution seemed the best way to attempt to represent the population as a whole and to examine the hypotheses proposed for this study.

After factoring, varimax rotation was used to achieve a factor matrix more closely meeting the criteria of simple structure. The rotated types account for 33%, 19%, 16%, 26%, and 7% (rounded percentages) respectively.

COMPILATION OF WEIGHTED TYPE ARRAYS

After rotation, PCQuanl produces a variety of type arrays that explains how each type is similar and different from all others. The statements for each type are listed from "most agreed with" to "least agreed with" to aid in interpretation. A Q type array "represents a hypothetical attitude, the 'common' attitude of the persons on the factor. The arrays are compiled from the total scores given the statement by all subjects on the factor, with each subject's statement scores weighted in accordance with his/her factor loading."[8]

INTERPRETATION OF Q TYPES

Interpretation of Q types has been called a "highly creative process."[9] The types are "operant combinations of 'like' people, i.e., combinations of people who have sorted items in similar, correlated, ways. The people are linked together by common beliefs, attitudes, opinions."[10]

Types are analyzed then by examining the attitudes that present themselves through the statement sortings. Additionally, subjects were asked to comment on the three statements with which they most strongly agree and on the three statements with which they most strongly disagree. Their comments provide insight into why they selected these statements or on how they are interpreting them.

Subjects also were asked to complete a questionnaire to obtain information about media habits, health status and demographics. In this case, responses to the questionnaire were entered into a computer program (CASES) and then analyzed using SPSS to examine each type in detail.

EXTENDING Q TYPES TO THE GENERAL POPULATION

One of the criticisms of Q methodology is that because it is a small sample technique, findings are not easily extended to the larger population. For example, because a Q type represents 35% of the total subjects completing Q sorts, there is no way of know if 35% of the total population belong to this type. Consequently, a second method has to be employed in order to determine the actual percent of the population a single Q type represents.

To overcome the difficulty with Q methodology, the author first administered and analyzed the Q sorts and then used the statements from the Q population in a telephone survey instrument, converting them to intensity scale items. Subjects were asked to rank each statement along a five-point scale (strongly agree to strongly disagree) rather than to rank each statement in relation to every other statement as subjects completing the Q sorts did.

Once the telephone survey data is collected, the next step is to match the respondents with the Q types found in the Q sort phase.

Matching the telephone survey results with the Q types proved no small task. Some of the difficulty resulted from the differences between being able to read the statements and ponder them, versus hearing the statements read (in random order) and reacting to each one individually. The subtleties of the Q sort rankings are difficult to retain. Also, a few of the statements had to be edited for the telephone survey because subjects have more trouble "hearing" a long statement than they have "reading" it for themselves. One statement was consistently misunderstood by subjects involved in the pre-test phase of the telephone survey. Because statement #11 (In health care promotions and advertising, white faces bringing bad news to blacks will not work.) was ranked in the neutral position (ranging from -.017 to .570) by all the Q types, this statement was dropped from the telephone instrument. Although no statement meanings were intentionally changed, it is likely that telephone subjects had more latitude for interpretation than did the Q sort subjects.

Several methods of matching the data from the two collections were attempted before a satisfactory solution was found. First, the statements that occupy the first four most-agree and the four-most-disagree positions in the Q sort arrays were used to create five clusters among the telephone respondents. The difficulty with this approach is that many of the same statements appear in prominent positions in different Q type arrays. Consequently, trying to determine which clusters matched the original types proved impossible. The next approach was to use the statements that were not necessarily at the top and bottom of the arrays, but which were identified as the most discriminating for identifying each type. (In other words, members of one type agree with the statement or disagreed with the statement more often than the members of the other types.) These clusters also proved impossible to match with the original arrays.

Finally, the best solution was obtained by treating each of the five types as if they are hypothetical subjects who participated in the telephone survey. The first step in accomplishing this is to convert the original z scores for each array into a five-point scale. For example, The Equalizers produced a z score of 1.85 for statement #24, 1.62 for statement #21, and 1.57 for statement #36. These statements occupy the +5 column on the Q sort grid.

The entire 11-column grid can be completed in this manner for each of the types.

Once the grid is completed, the results can be translated into a five-point scale. The statements in columns +4 and +5 become "strongly agree" responses on the scale, the ones in -4 and -5 become "strongly disagree" and so on.) The next step is to enter them into a data base alone with all the 527 telephone subjects as if they had responded to the statements by telephone.

Using SPSS the mean scores for these five "theoretical" persons are calculated. The means are then used to form the cluster centers for the telephone subject responses. This method made it possible to identify The Equalizers, The Adjusters, The Preventers, The Empathizers, and The Fixers easily. The SPSS cluster procedure obtains distance measures of similarities between or distances separating initial clusters based on the variable list (in this case the Q statements) provided. SPSS was asked to produce five clusters to correspond to each of the five Q types.

Discriminant analysis is used to check the cluster placement and to place into clusters subjects who had not responded to one or more of the Q statements in the telephone instrument. This procedure performs linear discriminant analysis for two or more groups (in this case, five groups). The results give a statistical probability for group membership in the cluster to which the subject initially has been assigned and also give the probability for membership in a second group. Also, if any subjects did not respond to one or more Q statements, discriminant analysis statistically assigns them to a group and gives the probability for that assignment. If there is high probability that the group to which the subjects were initially assigned is valid, the subjects are left in that cluster. If the probability is higher for an alternate group than for the initial group, subjects may be moved into a different cluster at that time. Subjects who initially are not placed in a cluster because of incomplete responses now can be placed in the cluster for which they have the highest probability score. Thus, all the randomly-selected telephone subjects, who represent the mass audience, can be clustered around the initial Q types obtained through a small sample technique. This overcomes perceived weaknesses in Q methodology and permits a more meaningful interpretation of the information obtained through random sampling methods.

It appears that three of the five telephone clusters match the Q types very closely. The other two do not match as closely, but they still show distinct differences in attitude from each other and the other clusters. Their general tendencies toward the statements (that is the tendency to agree with a statement or disagree with a statement) basically remains in tact.

Once each person's cluster membership is determined, the cluster numbers (1 through 5) are added to the telephone data set. Finally, individual cluster means are calculated for each statement. Significance is determined by subtracting the mean score for each cluster from the midpoint of the five-point scales (that is 3). If the difference is more than twice the standard error of the statement, the result is significant at the .05 level. If it is three times greater than the standard error, the result is significant at the .01 level.

In addition, crosstabulation tables are constructed using Pearson Chi-Square statistics to examine differences in demographics. A significance level of .05 is used to determine actual differences.

Most of the questions used in the supplemental questionnaire given to subjects completing the Q sorts are included in the telephone survey instrument. In addition to the 48 statements, the instrument contained questions about the subjects' media habits, their general health status and lifestyle changes, their opinion about universal insurance coverage, and their most frequent sources of health care information. Also, several demographic variables, such as gender and age, were included. Again, a few of the questions had to be altered for telephone administration. For example, rather than asking subjects to rank both the interpersonal and media sources of information from 1 to 10, they were read a list of interpersonal sources and asked for their No. 1 source. Then, they were read a list of media sources and asked for their No. 1 source.

TELEPHONE SURVEY METHODOLOGY

The final step in the data collection, the large-sample telephone survey, was conducted for the author by the Public Policy Research Center at the University of Missouri-St. Louis from June 13 to June 30, 1994.

A sample of telephone numbers roughly three times the desired N was generated at random using RMS software (developed by the Media Research Bureau, University of Missouri). Telephone exchanges were selected in St. Louis, Kansas City and Baton Rouge that would assure that about half the sample would be African American households. The Public Policy Research Center interviewers determined the age and race of each person before the interview took place in order to match the sample to U.S. Census data as closely as possible. A total of 527 persons were interviewed. Of these 208 are residents of St. Louis, 207 are residents of Kansas City, and 112 are residents of Baton Rouge, La. These three cities were selected because Kansas City and St. Louis contain the majority of the African American population in Missouri. Baton Rouge provides a smaller city setting and also adds the dimension of providing a Southern perspective. Also, Kansas City and St. Louis both have several black media, while Baton Rouge offers very little specialized media for the African American population.

Of the 527 persons interviewed, 49 percent are African American and 51 percent are Caucasian. Although this scheme under-represents the white population when suburban areas are included, it permits a large enough sample of both races to compare their responses. The results of this survey are discussed in Chapter VIII and Chapter IX.

NOTES

1. William Stephenson, foreword to *Political Subjectivity: Applications of Q Methodology in Political Science* by Steven R. Brown (New Haven: Yale University, 1980), ix-x.

2. Joye Patterson, "Attitudes About Science: A Dissection" (Ph.D. diss., University of Missouri, 1966), 30.

3. K. Knafl and M. Howard, "Interpreting and Reporting Qualitative Research," *Research in Nursing and Health*, 7, 17-24.

4. Ronald M. Weiers, *Marketing Research*, 2d. ed., (Englewood Cliffs, N.J.: Prentice Hall, 1988), 502.

5. Ibid., 502-503.

6. Gilbert A. Churchill Jr., *Marketing Research Methodological Foundations*, 4th ed., (Chicago: The Dryden Press, 1987), 770.

7. Brown, 40.

8. Keith P. Sanders, "On Interpretation of Q Factors," Handout for Advanced Research Methods class, November 1972, 2.

9. Ibid., 1.

10. Ibid., 2.

CHAPTER VII

Interpretation of the
Q Types

Five types from the factor analysis of the Q sorts have enough substance to be worthy of interpretation. The interpretations are based on 56 responses. All of the types—The Equalizers, The Preventers, The Empathizers, The Adjusters, and The Fixers—are analyzed below. (Total results for the Q sort participation quesionnaire appear in Appendix E, and results by factor appear in Appendix F.) It is important to note two of the types discussed are highly correlated (.825). This means that The Equalizers and The Adjusters could be subcategories of the same overall attitude, although the first type is predominately Caucasian and the second is primarily African American. Because of their similarities, these two types will be discussed first.

THE EQUALIZERS

The largest of the types with 22 subjects is The Equalizers. One subject has a negative factor loading (z-score). They see discrepancies in equal rights and access to health care, and they would like to see those discrepancies equalized. Comments collected from the subjects indicate a particular concern for the poor and disadvantaged in American society. Some obviously see the issue as an economic problem, while others focus more on access.

TABLE 3

DESCENDING ARRAY OF Z-SCORES AND ITEM
DESCRIPTIONS FOR THE EQUALIZERS

(Z-Scores of +/- .7 or Higher)

Statements	Z-Scores
(Agree)	
24. Lack of access to basic health care is an urgent issue currently troubling American society.	1.85
21. I believe that all Americans have a right—not a privilege— to health care.	1.62
36. Everyone does not have equal access to health care.	1.57
31. People are more likely to participate when they are recognized as a person, rather than labeled into minority groups.	1.48
38. Preventive health efforts must be improved in disadvantaged areas.	1.33
14. It is appropriate to use newspapers to try to get information out about health risks.	1.12
44. The whole health care delivery system needs to be overhauled.	1.11
13. If I felt by taking some precautions I could save myself money down the line I might take preventive measure to avoid that.	1.07
19. Physicians and health care practitioners need to respect the pride, values and folkways of people they are trying to reach.	.99
20. Community leaders are important to the success of any health care campaign.	.97
42. Rich people get better medical care than poor people.	.93
48. It doesn't matter to me whether doctors are black or white as long as they pay attention to my needs.	.82
23. Federal policies prohibiting discrimination in health service delivery should be enforced.	.81
27. To reach minority populations effectively with prevention information requires messages, programs tailored for a specific audience.	.80
8. Many people can't get health care because they have no transportation to a doctor's office, clinic, hospital.	.74
(Disagree)	
41. I will go to a doctor only if I think something is wrong with my health.	-.78
10. Getting the health care I need is usually too much trouble.	-1.00
30. Churches really have no role in promoting better physical health.	-1.02
45. I have a great deal of pride in the American health care system.	-1.03

TABLE 3 *(continued)*

Statements	Z-Scores
34. I know all I need to know about how to stay well.	-1.25
16. If I need medical care, I will most likely go to a hospital emergency room rather than to a private physician.	-1.30
43. My inclination is to stay away from doctors because you're not really sick until the doctor says you are.	-1.32
40. Racial barriers to health care are not an issue.	-1.35
7. There is not much I can do to keep from getting sick.	-1.49
17. Illness can be a punishment from God.	-1.50
33. Illnesses are not discussed in my family.	-1.60
6. I only need to worry about today because the future will take care of itself.	-1.65
5. We do not have a health care crisis in this country.	-1.97

Children and the elderly poor may be of special concern to this type. Above all, they want everyone to have a chance at equal access. Some comments provided by The Equalizers illustrate this attitude.

Statement:

24. Lack of access to basic health care is an urgent issue currently troubling American society.

Comments:

Too many people are not getting adequate health care.

Based on the fact that those who can pay get care; poor don't.

I feel it is an urgent need to access basic health care to many hard-working people who pay taxes and are unable to receive just the basic care needed to sustain a healthy life.

I agree with this because many people do not have access to health care that they need.

The children and older poor must be given preference in their health care. Our future depends on it.

Hard economic times compound the problem of health care for the disadvantaged.

Lack of health care is a major issue because the working class is the majority who lack it due to cost and who needs it most.

Health care is one of the basic issues in America.

People are dying every day because of a lack of health care.

The Equalizers strongly believe that lack of access to basic health care is an urgent issue—a crisis, in fact. Again, some blame economic factors while others see the spread of serious illnesses, such as AIDS, as the trigger. Lack of adequate insurance coverage also is mentioned.

Statement:

5.   We don't have a health care crisis in this country.

Comments:

Yes, we do—"big time"!

That is a complete untruth. It is so obvious that there is a crisis.

I disagree because everyone is not receiving proper medical treatment for reasons of economics. It should not be that way.

I strongly disagree that we don't have a health care crisis in this country because AIDS is affecting many; so is cancer and other dreadful diseases.

I disagree because there is a huge crisis dealing with health care in this country.

Cost of health care is increasing at alarming rate. Access to health care is uneven along racial lines.

Just look at the escalating costs and limited access for 40+ million people.

I've been out of work with no insurance after a cancer diagnosis. Getting state-of-the-art treatment is impossible.

There are too many people who will not seek medical attention because of no insurance.

To agree with this statement would deny that a problem exists in health care.

When people can't afford—or do not have the ability to pay—then we have a crisis.

The Equalizers think health care should be a right, not a privilege. However, they do not think that everyone in America currently has that right because of economics, lack of access, or race.

Statement:

21. I believe that *all* Americans have a right—not a privilege—to health care.

Comments:

All Americans—not just those that can afford it.

I believe we should be able to take care of our own.

Each person must have proper health care in order to protect our society. (The spreading of diseases.)

As a cancer survivor, I deplore any form of discrimination based on economics or health history.

As a minority physician who has been around, I feel strongly it should be a right.

I think every human being should have the right to receive health care.

I agree with this because it shouldn't be a privilege to be well, it should be a right.

I truly believe all Americans have a right; God said all men are created equal.

Access is another important issue to The Equalizers. They strongly believe that not everyone has access, often because of economic difficulties or location.

Statement:

36. Everyone does *not* have equal access to health care.

Comments:

It depends on who can afford care—if you don't have insurance or $—no care!

Because the way health care is structured now people just don't have access.

It is a true statement. Economics and race play an important role in health care not being equal.

The poor and rural people have less access.

Having spent a year in south central LA in a county hospital (as a physician), I saw the difference in support.

It is true that everyone doesn't have equal access to health care because of poor transportation, poor housing, and too many homeless.

Health care is not disbursed among the young and elderly and minority population.

If everyone had equal care there would be no need to be concerned about our health care program.

It is a true statement. Economics and race play an important role in health care being equal.

The Equalizers also are concerned about racism standing in the way of equity in health care.

Statement:

40.   Racial barriers to health care are *not* an issue.

Comments:

Race will always be an issue until people let go of prejudices and think of how you would want to be treated. And (doctors are) willing to practice in black communities.

People expect most blacks to be treated as indigents. They assume they cannot understand what is happening to them. Untrue!

Racism is a barrier to good health care; just look into a ghetto anywhere in the U.S.

The statement is not true because it is mostly minorities that have a problem with affording health care.

The Equalizers care about the way people are treated. They think people are more likely to participate (in the health care system) if they are recognized as persons rather than labeled into minority groups. They expect physicians and health care practitioners to respect the culture of the people they are trying to reach.

Statement:

31.   People are more likely to participate when they are recognized as a person, rather than being labeled, isolated and separated into minority groups.

Comments:

We often label people and stereotypes and then look down on them acting as if we are their holy saviors. We must stop all the labeling and recognize people as persons.

People do not and cannot learn unless they feel they are important.

People should not be labeled or placed into groups.

If a person is treated as a person instead of a number.

Because they are concerned with racism, access, and the respect with which people are treated, The Equalizers want efforts made to improve health care in disadvantaged areas.

Statement:

38. Preventive health efforts must be improved in disadvantaged areas.

Comments:

For all the same reasons. (Because some minorities may not have access to newspapers or TV and reading level may not be on level literature is distributed.)

It is a very true statement. Most health care services are not located in disadvantaged areas.

The Equalizers strongly disagree that they only need to worry about today because tomorrow will take care of itself.

Statement:

6. The future will take care of itself; I only need to worry about today.

Comment:

You need to worry about the future in order to live a long life!

Individuals must act now to address health care issues. The cost of the system will soon "break the bank."

An ounce of prevention is worth a pound of cure.

This attitude is part of the reason so many people are unhealthy.

I don't believe in this statement.

There also is a strong belief among The Equalizers that individuals do have some control over their own health, although the subjects may not believe they have all the knowledge they need. (On the accompanying questionnaire, about 14% indicated they have not made any recent lifestyle changes to improve either their own or their family's health. None said they had quit smoking—although this particular questionnaire did not determine if they were currently smoking—and only one person had reduced alcohol intake. By contrast, 77% said they had modified their diets, almost 41% had increased the amount they exercise, and 14% had made other lifestyles changes (such as reducing stress, relaxing more, etc.).

They do not view illness as a punishment from God, and they think there are steps they can take to keep from getting ill.

Statement:

7.   There is not much I can do to keep from getting sick.

Comments:

Health information and prevention is very important.

We are in control of most health problems. Eating properly, exercising, also dressing appropriately.

Statement:

17.   Illness can be a punishment from God.

Comments:

I do not feel God punishes you with illness. God is not a vengeful God. Illness could be the result of many things, i.e., liver damage from alcohol and drugs.

God does not punish in this way—we often bring illness by our habits and carelessness.

I think there are mystical qualities to illness—but not this one.

Has nothing to do with religious beliefs. It depends on how your lifestyle is!

I believe that God is a loving God, and random illness is just not the way God works.

An illness is not given to us by God because we deserve it. This is totally untrue.

No punishment is of God.

As a scientist and a physician (I know) illness has a cause and can be precipitated by numerous factors.

I also strongly disagree that illness is punishment from God because Jesus came to make us free from sickness and God doesn't have to punish us with illnesses. He's God and can punish us any way he wants to.

Just another excuse to elude responsibility for oneself.

In addition, The Equalizers are willing to discuss illnesses with other family members, often doing so on a regular basis. .

Statement:

33. Illnesses are not discussed in my family.

Comments:

Illnesses are always discussed in my family because it directly affects me and my lifestyle.

My family discusses *all* health problems.

Illnesses are always discussed in my family. We learn or hear of a lot of illnesses.

We talk about health always.

We discuss health care almost daily.

The Equalizers' sorting of other statements indicate they will go to a doctor for checkups or when they are sick and are more likely to choose a private doctor or clinic rather than go to a hospital emergency room. They generally do not think getting the health care they need is too much trouble, although they do see lack of transportation to a doctor's office, clinic, or hospital as a major barrier to health care for some.

The Equalizers are willing to take health precautions or preventive actions if it might save them money down the line. They do not care about the race of their physicians as long as they pay attention to their needs. Also, they are likely to go to a doctor for a routine checkup rather than wait until they are not feeling well. (Ninety-one percent have seen their doctors in the past year.)

Because of inequality in access, The Equalizers tend to believe the entire health care system needs to be overhauled. Consequently, they lack pride in the American health care system. The Equalizers see two predominant reasons for unequal care. One is that the rich receive better care than the poor. Going along with this is the belief that federal policies prohibiting discrimination in health service delivery should be enforced. They do not believe that inequality occurs either because minorities have not been taught how to use the health care system or because physicians are prejudiced against African Americans. The Equalizers doubt that African Americans are reluctant to seek early treatment for illness because care is provided by white medical personnel. They also do not think the media care more about diseases that affect whites and ignore diseases that affect African Americans.

The Equalizers believe that to reach minority populations effectively, prevention messages and programs should be tailored for and targeted toward a specific audience. They see newspapers as the main way to get information out about health risks, although they also tend to read health stories in both newspapers and magazines and think television can carry important messages. They also view community leaders and churches as important to the success of a health care campaign. Not surprisingly, The Equalizers are among the lightest television viewers with 32% watching from two to ten hours a week and 32% watching from 11 to 20 hours per week.

Almost 96% read newspapers regularly, with 41% reading at least one African American newspaper. Also, The Equalizers are the most trusting of the information in the health articles they read. Fifty-nine percent said they generally believe the information, while 23% said the source of the article is important to their evaluation, and only 18% said they usually question the information.

When asked about their knowledge of Pres. Clinton's health plan on the questionnaire, only one person (a physician) claimed to be knowledgeable. However, 59% said they had read or heard something about the plan, 27% claimed limited knowledge and 9% (two persons) said they know nothing about the plan. Even so, people in this type are the most likely to give some support to Clinton's plan, with 27% supporting it outright and 18% saying they liked some aspects and disliked others. However, they are pessimistic that a health care system that gives everyone the help they need is possible.

The subjects forming this type are 59% African American and 36% white. The one lone Hispanic in the P sample also is in this type. This group then is the most diverse in terms of race and income, but they are generally more highly educated than the rest of the P sample. They are trusting of their sources of health information, but this may be in part because they rely on medical personnel and medical-related publications more than the popular press for their information. They do not seem to be personally cut off from health care services, nor do they lack insurance or other means of paying for health care for the most part.

Although they may discuss health issues with family and friends, The Equalizers do not consider these people to be major sources of health information. They also are generally healthy, and they think everyone—regardless of race or economic status—has a right to be equally healthy and to have equal access to the health care system. They are strongly convinced that access is not equal, and they want the system overhauled. This may explain some of the support for the Clinton plan, even though they do not have much knowledge of the specific components of that plan. A table comparing demographic information for each type appears in Appendix F.

THE ADJUSTERS

The second largest type with 15 members is The Adjusters. It is a predominately African American type (80%) and is the most "male" of any type (60%). They believe that health care is most available to those who have the means to pay for it, and that education is the key to improving the general health of the population. They are less likely than The Equalizers to think the entire health care system needs to be overhauled. Rather they would prefer to "adjust" the system, rather than to move to an entirely new system.

TABLE 4

**DESCENDING ARRAY OF Z-SCORES AND
ITEM DESCRIPTIONS FOR THE ADJUSTERS**

(Z-Scores of +/- .7 or Higher)

Statements	Z-Scores
(Agree)	
36. Everyone does not have equal access to health care.	1.92
42. Rich people get better medical care than poor people.	1.91
21. I believe that all Americans have a right—not a privilege— to health care.	1.74
38. Preventive health efforts must be improved in disadvantaged areas.	1.40
24. Lack of access to basic health care is an urgent issue currently troubling American society.	1.35
29. Access to health care and to the means of maintaining health are simply out of the reach of those not able to pay.	1.16
48. It doesn't matter to me whether doctors are black or white as long as they pay attention to my needs.	1.08
3. Blacks are the victims of an economic system that dictates both their ability to receive health services, quality of health.	1.06
4. Support groups are important because many people can relate to others who are like themselves.	1.00
20. Community leaders are important to the success of any health care campaign.	.97
23. Federal policies prohibiting discrimination in health service delivery should be enforced.	.92
49. As long as a disease is hitting white people, the media care. But if it's hitting mainly Blacks, they don't worry about it too much.	.89
27. To reach minority populations effectively with prevention information requires messages, programs tailored for a specific audience.	.76
(Disagree)	
40. Racial barriers to health care are not an issue.	-.98
33. Illnesses are not discussed in my family.	-1.08
30. Churches really have not role in promoting better physical health.	-1.10
16. If I need medical care, I will most likely go to a hospital emergency room rather than to a private physician.	-1.12
10. Getting the health care I need is usually too much trouble.	-1.16
2. Doctors are prejudiced against Blacks.	-1.22

TABLE 4 *(continued)*

Statements	Z-Scores
43. My inclination is to stay away from doctors because you're not really sick until the doctor says you are.	-1.26
5. We do not have a health care crisis in this country.	-1.38
6. I only need to worry about today because the future will take care of itself.	-1.42
34. I know all I need to know about how to stay well.	-1.49
1. Blacks are reluctant to obtain early treatment for illnesses because care is provided by white medical personnel.	-1.64
17. Illness can be a punishment from God.	-1.78
7. There is not much I can do to keep from getting sick.	-1.89

First, The Adjusters strongly agree that not everyone has equal access to health care mostly because of economics rather than racism. They are concerned with people who fall through the cracks of the present system:

Statement:

36. Everyone does *not* have equal access to health care.

Comment:

Many people fall in the middle—not poor enough for Medicaid, not rich enough for private care.

Homeless, unemployed transients are denied basic care.

I feel that is the problem with the health care system. If everyone had access as well as adequate health care, then there wouldn't be such a big problem.

Some people who cannot be classified as indigent and not eligible for insurance do not have the same access to health care as others.

The Adjusters are partly distinguished from the other types by their attitude toward the reason for inequity in access. They strongly believe economics are at the heart of the problem. Rich people simply get better medical care than poor people. They believe access to health care and to the means of maintaining health are out of the reach of those not able to pay.

Statement:

42. Rich people get better medical care than poor people.

Comment:

The rich have access to the newest techniques—sometimes not covered by insurance.

Quality costs, and quality is difficult to find today.

Health care is expensive and those with the money can afford insurance.

All three statements (#3, #29, #42) reflect my firm belief that poverty is the number one cause of major illness in this country.

Rich people can afford good medical care whenever they want it.

You get what you paid for.

Quality costs, and quality is difficult to find today.

The Adjusters, like The Equalizers, believe that all Americans have a right to health care. In fact, they are the most likely of all the types to believe this.

Statement:

21. I believe that all Americans have a right—not a privilege—to health care.

Comment:

Something should be done to protect the health of all citizens, even those who can't afford it.

I believe that *all* Americans have (this) right.

Health care should not be like a driver's permit.

(I agree with) the word "all."

I believe that all Americans have a right to health care, no matter what gender, race, etc.

Something should be done to protect health of all citizens, even those who can't afford it.

It is my opinion that every American (rich or poor) has a right to good health care.

The right to life, liberty and the pursuit of happiness includes access to all resources.

By tieing these three statements together (#21, #24, #44), I'll say that I believe every American citizen has a right to be cured of any illness that is curable through access to a basic health care facility. As our system stands now, that is not the case for many poor citizens. Therefore the system needs an overhaul.

More than any other type, The Adjusters believe that African Americans are the victims of the American economic system. Also, they are the most likely to believe that minorities have not been taught how to use the health care system. Consequently, members of this type believe that preventive health efforts must be improved in disadvantaged areas.

Statement:

38. Preventive health efforts must be improved in disadvantaged areas.

Comment:

Blacks die and suffer unnecessarily because preventive health is not practiced.

They agree that lack of access to basic health care is an urgent issue currently troubling American society.

Statement:

24. Lack of access to basic health care is an urgent issue currently troubling American society.

Comment:

Preventive health care, care for minor illness, ignored in favor of larger issues.

The Adjusters do not care whether their doctors are black or white, and they doubt that doctors are prejudiced against blacks or that African Americans are reluctant to seek treatment from nonblack medical personnel.

Statement:

1. Blacks are reluctant to obtain early treatment for illnesses because care is provided by nonblack medical personnel.

Comments:

Black people I know don't mind white or non-black physicians.

This is usually the lesser of the reasons for Blacks not obtaining early treatment.

The Adjusters strongly disagree that there is not much they can do to keep from getting sick, although they are more likely than The Equalizers to view this as a matter of education rather than a matter of personal action.

(They, personally, doubt they have enough information about how to stay well.)

Statement:

7.   There is not much I can do to keep from getting sick.

Comments:

All three statements (#7, #17, #6) reflect a view that illness cannot be effectively fought. This goes against everything I believe as a physician.

I believe education is the key to health care. We must understand what makes us ill. The health care was built for the wealthy. No money, no care. We have a health care crisis in minority areas only.

I believe that an individual has a lot of control over their health and if they can control it, then they can reduce the chances of getting sick.

Remember: (An ounce of) prevention is worth. . . .

(Only one person in this type has not made recent lifestyle changes to improve their health or the health of their families. One person had quit smoking, 12 of 15 had modified their diets, six of 15 had increased their exercise, four of 15 had made other changes.)

They also do not think illness is a punishment from God. However, The Adjusters view a belief in God's punishment as illogical or superstitious. The Equalizers, on the other hand, view God as benevolent and caring rather than punishing.

Statement:

17.   Illness can be a punishment from God.

Comments:

This is a superstitious belief. No basis in fact or reality.

Hogwash!

Myth.

If God punishes with ill health, then why are innocent infants sick? What did they do wrong?

There is a health care crisis in The Adjusters' view, although they may see lack of insurance and gaps in coverage (elements which can be adjusted) as more of a problem than the proliferation of AIDS or other serious diseases.

Statement:

5.   We don't have a health care crisis in this country.

Comment:

This statement is false because we have millions of people not covered by insurance.

When you look at our different systems and still some people don't fall into any one—there is a crisis (for the number is getting larger).

They do not personally feel that the current health care system makes them feel poor, and they do not believe that hospital personnel make people wait longer if they do not have insurance.

The Adjusters do believe that racial barriers to health care are important issues. Along with this, they believe federal policies prohibiting discrimination in health service delivery should be enforced. They are more hopeful than The Equalizers that a health care system that gives everyone the help they need is possible.

The Adjusters are more likely than The Equalizers to think support groups are important because many people can relate to others who are like themselves. Unlike The Equalizers, The Adjusters do not think that people are more likely to participate when they are recognized as a person rather than as a minority. They agree with The Equalizers that community leaders are important to the success of any health care campaign and that churches have a role in promoting better physical health. They think, in order to reach minority populations effectively with prevention information messages, programs tailored for a specific audience are required. (They prefer adjustments in current messages, rather than specifically targeting groups of people.)

However, The Adjusters, unlike The Equalizers, do not think newspapers are an effective means of providing information about health risks although they probably do read newspaper and magazine articles about health. (In fact, The Adjusters are the most likely to regularly read health care articles. Sixty percent regularly read them, 33% occasionally read them, and only one person doesn't read them. Fifty-three percent generally believe the articles, 27% usually question them, and 20% said their belief depends on the article source.) They are more likely to think television is an effective medium for health care messages. (One-third watch television from two to ten hours a week, 20% watch 11 to 20 hours, 40% watch 21 to 30 hours, and 7% watch from 31 to 72 hours per week. Ninety-three percent read newspapers, and 73% read at least one black newspaper.)

Unlike The Equalizers, The Adjusters think the media care more about diseases that affect white people than they do about diseases that affect African Americans. (Because so many subjects in this type are African American, they may simply believe much of the media are not very relevant to them personally.)

They also think it is important to consider the future rather than just worrying about today. Getting the health care they need is usually not too much trouble.

The Adjusters may be less likely than The Equalizers to discuss illnesses with other family members. They personally have no inclination to stay away from doctors, and they are not likely to use a hospital emergency room rather than to go to a private physician.

The Adjusters are less likely than The Equalizers to take preventive health measure to save themselves money down the line, and they are less certain that lack of transportation is an important barrier to health care.

They are more optimistic than The Equalizers that a health care system that gives everyone the help they need is possible.

Twenty percent said they are knowledgeable about the Clinton health care plan, while 60% have heard or read something about it, 13% have limited knowledge, and 7% know nothing about the plan. Almost 27% support Clinton's plan, 13% oppose it, 27% think the plan is too complicated to understand, 27% have no opinion and one person supports some aspects and opposes others.

In some ways, The Adjusters are the most "middle" of the types. Members tend to be middle age and middle class. They understand that health care barriers prevent access for many people, but they probably do not identify with lack of health care as much as The Empathizers.

THE OBLIVIOUS PREVENTERS

Although The Equalizers cut across racial lines and The Adjusters are predominantly African American, the eleven subjects who form The Oblivious Preventers type are primarily white Americans. Although they share areas of agreement with the previous two groups, The Preventers differ in important ways. They believe that it is important to avail oneself of medical intervention and to use community programs and health campaigns to encourage health. Unlike The Equalizers and The Adjusters, they express pride in the American health care system. Additionally, they appear oblivious to any racial barriers that might stand in the way of good health.

The Preventers don't care about their physicians' race as long as they pay attention to their personal needs.

TABLE 5
DESCENDING ARRAY OF Z-SCORES AND ITEM DESCRIPTIONS FOR THE OBLIVIOUS PREVENTERS
(Z-Scores of +/- .7 or Higher)

Statements	Z-Scores
(Agree)	
48. It doesn't matter to me whether doctors are black or white as long as they pay attention to my needs.	1.95
19. Physicians and health care practitioners need to respect the pride, values and folkways of people they are trying to reach.	1.90
38. Preventive health efforts must be improved in disadvantaged areas.	1.62
31. People are more likely to participate when they are recognized as a person, rather than labeled into minority groups.	1.62
20. Community leaders are important to the success of any health care campaign.	1.34
22. If I'm not feeling well, I have no trouble finding time to go to the doctor.	1.24
4. Support groups are important because many people can relate to others who are like themselves.	1.17
13. If I felt by taking some precautions I could save myself money down the line I might take preventive measure to avoid that.	1.15
45. I have a great deal of pride in the American health care system.	1.14
37. I take the time to read health stories in newspapers and magazines.	1.06
15. If you have an important message about health care, put it on television.	.98
27. To reach minority populations effectively with prevention information requires messages, programs tailored for a specific audience.	.98
14. It is appropriate to use newspapers to try to get information out about health risks.	.91
25. Any successful health campaign that could change behaviors would originate in my community rather than at the state, national level.	.84
36. Everyone does not have equal access to health care.	.70

TABLE 5 *(continued)*

Statements	Z-Scores
(Disagree)	
18. The health care system makes me feel like I'm poor.	-.72
6. I only need to worry about today because the future will take care of itself.	-.77
8. Many people can't get health care because they have no transportation to a doctor's office, clinic, hospital.	-.87
43. My inclination is to stay away from doctors because you're not really sick until the doctor says you are.	-.93
47. The ultimate solution to providing adequate health care for Blacks is to educate enough black health care providers.	-1.09
29. Access to health care and to the means of maintaining health are simply out of the reach of those not able to pay.	-1.10
16. If I need medical care, I will most likely go to a hospital emergency room rather than to a private physician.	-1.22
39. The federal government's health policies are geared for the general population. They don't help minorities very much.	-1.27
1. Blacks are reluctant to obtain early treatment for illnesses because care is provided by white medical personnel.	-1.28
7. There is not much I can do to keep from getting sick.	-1.28
2. Doctors are prejudiced against Blacks.	-1.43
17. Illness can be a punishment from God.	-1.48
3. Blacks are the victims of an economic system that dictates both their ability to receive health services, quality of health.	-1.58
49. As long as a disease is hitting white people, the media care. But if it's hitting mainly Blacks, they don't worry about it too much.	-1.58

Statement:

48. It doesn't matter to me whether doctors are black or white as long as they pay attention to my needs.

Comment:

I know many doctors—race is not an important issue.

I select a provider based upon qualifications, interest in me and my family and not the color of their skin.

The most important thing is that a doctor gives his best to his patients.

I want my doctor (any doctor) to help me if I'm hurt—they've all had training—the same.

Going along with this attitude, they strongly agree that physicians and health care practitioners need to respect the pride, values, and folkways of the people (likely regardless of race) they are trying to reach.

Statement:

19. Physicians and health care practitioners need to respect the pride, values, and folkways of people they are trying to reach.

Comment:

Everyone needs to respect the next person more in all aspects.

Everyone is not alike.

The Preventers show other signs of taking their personal health seriously. If they are not feeling well, they have no trouble finding the time to go to a doctor. They have no inclination to stay away from doctors, and they are likely to go to a personal physician or clinic rather than to an emergency room for care.

The Preventers are likely to take precautions or preventive actions to save money on health care down the line and indicate a concern for the future. They take the time to read newspaper and magazine health stories. Finally, they think support groups are important.

The third most agreed with statement is that preventive health efforts must be improved in disadvantaged areas.

Statement:

38. Preventive health efforts must be improved in disadvantaged areas.

Comment:

Disadvantaged areas have neither the resources in education to practice preventive medicine.

Providing better living conditions to the disadvantaged will improve health matters.

They believe people are more likely to participate when they are recognized as individuals rather than stereotyped.

Statement:

31. People are more likely to participate when they are recognized as a person, rather than being labeled, isolated, and separated into minority groups.

Comment:

If people feel like a number instead of a person, they will not participate.

I am a person, and I do not like the idea of labeling people.

Medical care cannot be given on a racial/ethnic basis—only individual.

Other statements also reveal a sense of community among The Preventers. They see local leaders as very important to the success of any health care campaign, and they agree to a lesser extent that any successful health campaign that could change behaviors would have to originate in the community rather than at the state or national level.

Statement:

20. Community leaders are important to the success of any health care campaign.

Comment:

Because these leaders have the skills, knowledge, love, and understanding for anybody.

The Preventers consider television the medium for important health care messages, but they also think newspapers are an appropriate vehicle for health care information. They think to reach minority populations effectively with prevention information requires messages and programs tailored for a specific audience.

They concede somewhat that not everyone has equal access to health care. Otherwise, though, they show little agreement that racial barriers and/or discrimination in the health care system exists.

For example, they strongly disagree that the media only care when a disease is affecting white people and ignore the disease if it is predominately affecting black people.

Statement:

49. As long as a disease is hitting white people, the media care. But if it's hitting black people, they are not going to worry about it too much.

Comment:

I have not observed this to be true.

The statement is not true and is of a prejudiced nature.

I disagree because it is not a true statement.

They equally disagree that blacks are the victims of an economic system that dictates both their ability to receive health services and quality of health.

Statement:

3. Blacks are the victims of an economic system that dictates both their ability to receive health services and quality of health care.

Comment:

They aren't victims of anything.

I do not believe this is so in this area.

The Preventers are much more likely to blame lifestyles, rather than God, for illness.

Statement:

17. Illness can be a punishment from God.

Comments:

Anyone who believes in God cannot believe this statement.

God does not punish with illness.

God doesn't choose to hurt us. We bring illness and disease when we sin. We bring it on us.

I believe that clean living helps in life.

Statement:

7.   There is not much I can do to keep from getting sick.

Comments:

I believe there is plenty I can do to prevent illness.

Many lifestyles decisions affect our health.

They also disagreed with other statements that said doctors are prejudiced against blacks, that blacks are reluctant to obtain early treatment of illnesses because care is provided by white medical personnel, that the ultimate solution to providing adequate health care for blacks is to educate enough black health care providers, and that the federal government's health policies are geared for the general population and do not help minorities.

Statement:

2.   Doctors are prejudiced against blacks.

Comments:

The statement simply is not true.

Medical training precludes racial bias. Each individual is unique.

Not true.

A general statement. Some doctors may be, others are not.

They also dismiss other potential barriers to health care. They disagree that access to health care and to the means of maintaining health are out of the reach of those not able to pay and that many people can't get health care because they have no transportation to a doctor's office, clinic, or hospital. Finally, they disagree that the health care system makes them feel like they are poor. However, they doubt that a health care system that gives all citizens the help they need is possible.

Almost 55% of The Preventers regularly read health articles in newspapers and magazines, while 36% read them occasionally, and 9% rarely or never read them. Among the types, The Preventers are the most questioning of the information in the health articles they read. Six of the eleven said they evaluate the information, usually by source, before deciding whether to believe it. Only one person in this type said he believes the information, while 36% usually question its accuracy.

The Preventers are much less likely than The Equalizers to have seen a physician in the past year (73%), but 18% had personally been hospitalized, while 36% said family members had been hospitalized. Almost 91% of The Preventers said they have family physicians.

When asked about their knowledge of Pres. Clinton's health plan, 36% (four persons) claimed to be knowledgeable, while 36% said they had read or heard something about the plan, and 27% claimed limited knowledge. Only one person supports Clinton's plan, while three oppose it, three think it is too complicated to understand, and three expressed reservations about it but stopped short of either supporting or opposing it.

THE EMPATHIZERS

This type contains only four people, all of whom are African American with low household incomes. The type is labeled "The Empathizers" because the subjects exhibit an understanding for the concerns of many African Americans and the poor. They may, in fact, empathize because they *are* the African American poor.

However, The Empathizers also agree that the media care more about disease if it is affecting white rather than black people and that if a message is labeled as a black health care concern, white people will dismiss it.

Statement:

49. As long as a disease is hitting white people, the media care. But if it's hitting black people, they are not going to worry about it too much.

Comments:

Just look at TV and you will see how the media do about disease of white people.

This is a strong statement. It happens each and every day.

TABLE 6
DESCENDING ARRAY OF Z-SCORES AND ITEM
DESCRIPTIONS FOR THE EMPATHIZERS
(Z-Scores of +/- .7 or Higher)

Statements	Z-Scores
(Agree)	
48. It doesn't matter to me whether doctors are black or white as long as they pay attention to my needs.	1.96
49. As long as a disease is hitting white people, the media care. But if it's hitting mainly Blacks, they don't worry about it too much.	1.94
31. People are more likely to participate when they are recognized as a person, rather than labeled into minority groups.	1.92
42. Rich people get better medical care than poor people.	1.70
35. If you go to a hospital and they figure you may not have insurance or you're undercovered, they always make you wait.	1.37
9. It is more important for an American health care system to give free medical care to the poor than to middle, upper income.	1.33
32. The ability of a doctor to help me depends in large part on my belief that the doctor will help me.	1.32
26. If you label the message as a black health care concern, then white people will say "that's for Blacks" right away.	1.26
23. Federal policies prohibiting discrimination in health service delivery should be enforced.	1.02
21. I believe that all Americans have a right—not a privilege— to health care.	.90
(Disagree)	
27. To reach minority populations effectively with prevention information requires messages, programs tailored for a specific audience.	-.73
7. There is not much I can do to keep from getting sick.	-.74
17. Illness can be a punishment from God.	-.74
8. Many people can't get health care because they have no transportation to a doctor's office, clinic, hospital.	-.77
34. I know all I need to know about how to stay well.	-.82
16. If I need medical care, I will most likely go to a hospital emergency room rather than to a private physician.	-.85
14. It is appropriate to use newspapers to try to get information out about health risks.	-1.05
1. Blacks are reluctant to obtain early treatment for illnesses because care is provided by white medical personnel.	-1.07
33. Illnesses are not discussed in my family.	-1.24
45. I have a great deal of pride in the American health care system.	-1.37

TABLE 6 *(continued)*

Statements	Z-Scores
10. Getting the health care I need is usually too much trouble.	-1.40
46. Minorities have not been taught how to use the health care system.	-1.43
5. We do not have a health care crisis in this country.	-1.72
12. The real key to good health is to lead a clean, moral life.	-1.77
47. The ultimate solution to providing adequate health care for Blacks is to educate enough black health care providers.	-2.11

Furthermore, they think people are more likely to participate when they are recognized as an individual rather than as a minority .

Statement:

31. People are more likely to participate when they are recognized as a person rather than labeled into minority groups.

Comments:

We have different color skin, but we are all the same under this skin.

You can't judge a book by its cover.

The Empathizers believe that rich people get better medical care than poor people perhaps not because they can afford better care but because the wealthy do not have to deal with government programs.

Statement:

42. Rich people get better medical care than poor people.

Comment:

Because rich people are not on Medicare and Medicaid.

The Empathizers agree that patients have to wait for care if hospital personnel think a potential patient is uninsured.

Statement:

35. If you go to a hospital and they figure you may not have insurance or you're undercovered, they always make you wait. But, if you have insurance, they take you right in there because they know they are going to get their money.

Comments:

I have seen this happen, and I strongly agree with the statement.

They believe there is a health care crisis in America, and they lack pride in the health care system. Additionally, they believe it is more important for an American health care system to give free medical care to the poor than to middle and upper income people and that federal policies prohibiting discrimination in health service delivery should be enforced.

Statement:

5. We do not have a health care crisis in this country.

Comment:

We do with all the new, different things coming out now.

We really do have a health care crisis.

They disagree that minorities have not been taught how to use the health care system, or that reaching a minority population requires messages and programs tailored for a specific audience.

Statement:

46. Minorities have not been taught how to use the health care system.

Comment:

That's not right. A lot of blacks know how to deal with it.

Interestingly, the statement they most disagree with is that the ultimate solution to providing adequate health care for blacks is to education enough black health care providers.

Statement:

47. The ultimate solution to providing adequate health care for black people is to educate enough black health care providers to do it.

Comments:

We do not need black doctors for blacks and white doctors for whites.

Health care for black people can be provided adequate from any body as long as he/she knows how to provide it.

Doctors are doctors; all of them should care about their patients.

The Empathizers disagree that the real key to good health is to lead a clean, moral life, and they tend not to believe that illness is a punishment from God.

Statement:

12. The real key to good health is to lead a clean, moral life.

Comment:

You can lead a clean and moral life and still get sick.

They are not likely to go to an emergency room for routine medical care, or to think that getting health care is too much trouble.

Statement:

10. Getting the health care I need is usually too much trouble.

Comment:

You can always find a way to get to the doctor, hospital, etc.

The Empathizers do discuss illnesses with family members, and they somewhat believe that they do not have all the information they need about how to stay well. They also agree that the ability of a doctor to help them depends in part on their belief that the physician will help them.

This group tends not to be very concerned with media messages or community-oriented programs. They disagree that it is appropriate to use newspapers to try to get information out about health risks. (In fact, none said they generally believe the health articles they read.) Consequently, of all the types this one may be the most difficult to reach through media health campaigns.

In summary, this group perhaps best typifies the low income African American. They do not seem to be in particularly good health, yet they have had very little recent contact with the health care system. They are quite sensitive to the problems of race and poverty, but they certainly do not blame the problems on the lack of trained, black health care providers. They also do not dwell on any barrier to health care except poverty. They seem to neither agree or disagree that a health care system that gives everyone the help they need is possible.

The Empathizers are much less likely than the other two types to believe they have control over illness, even though they have made lifestyle changes toward that end. In accordance with the knowledge gap hypothesis, they do indicate they lack knowledge about health care and are the least likely to have any information about the Clinton health plan. Also, although all said they read newspapers, they are likely more dependent on the electronic media for information and entertainment.

THE FIXERS

The fifth and final type is also very small (four subjects). It is worth describing for three reasons. First, this is the only type that believes (somewhat) that illness can be a punishment from God. Second, they strongly disagree that they know all they need to know about how to stay well. They also seem to think that government policies are benefitting minorities, even though they have no pride in the American health care system.

This type is named "The Fixers" because its members show traits of seeing problems and wanting to rectify them. For example, they believe equal access to health care is not a reality.

Statement:

36. Everyone does not have equal access to health care.

Comments:

The distribution of medical resources has nothing to do with the distribution of need, i.e. health care in rural areas.

Routine care is often too expensive for the poor!!

However, the next statement they most agree with is that preventive health efforts must be improved in disadvantaged areas.

Statement:

38. Preventive health efforts must be improved in disadvantaged areas.

Comment:

Unless we prevent more illnesses, there is not enough money to fix people after their health is broken.

(It is) more economical to prevent disease than treat once it occurs.

TABLE 7
DESCENDING ARRAY OF Z-SCORES AND ITEM DESCRIPTIONS FOR THE FIXERS
(Z-Scores of +/- .7 or Higher)

Statements	Z-Scores
(Agree)	
36. Everyone does not have equal access to health care.	2.22
38. Preventive health efforts must be improved in disadvantaged areas.	2.22
23. Federal policies prohibiting discrimination in health service delivery should be enforced.	1.40
21. I believe that all Americans have a right—not a privilege—to health care.	1.37
27. To reach minority populations effectively with prevention information requires messages, programs tailored for a specific audience.	1.31
42. Rich people get better medical care than poor people.	1.19
31. People are more likely to participate when they are recognized as a person, rather than labeled into minority groups.	1.08
32. The ability of a doctor to help me depends in large part on my belief that the doctor will help me.	.96
24. Lack of access to basic health care is an urgent issue currently troubling American society.	.94
35. If you go to a hospital and they figure you may not have insurance or you're undercovered, they always make you wait.	.89
48. It doesn't matter to me whether doctors are black or white as long as they pay attention to my needs.	.88

TABLE 7 *(continued)*

Statements	Z-Scores
25. Any successful health campaign that could change behaviors would originate in my community rather than at the state, national level.	.87
17. Illness can be a punishment from God.	.86
19. Physicians and health care practitioners need to respect the pride, values and folkways of people they are trying to reach.	.77
(Disagree)	
12. The real key to good health is to lead a clean, moral life.	-.72
2. Doctors are prejudiced against Blacks.	-.76
22. If I'm not feeling well, I have no trouble finding time to go to the doctor.	-.77
10. Getting the health care I need is usually too much trouble.	-.80
1. Blacks are reluctant to obtain early treatment for illnesses because care is provided by white medical personnel.	-1.02
9. It is more important for an American health care system to give free medical care to the poor than to middle, upper income.	-1.15
45. I have a great deal of pride in the American health care system.	-1.26
39. The federal government's health policies are geared for the general population. They don't help minorities very much.	-1.30
8. Many people can't get health care because they have no transportation to a doctor's office, clinic, hospital.	-1.35
5. We do not have a health care crisis in this country.	-1.42
16. If I need medical care, I will most likely go to a hospital emergency room rather than to a private physician.	-1.48
6. I only need to worry about today because the future will take care of itself.	-1.59
7. There is not much I can do to keep from getting sick.	-1.74
34. I know all I need to know about how to stay well.	-1.81

Every one of The Fixers ranked statements #36 and #38 either +5 or +4. In their opinion providing equal access to medical care obviously must begin in disadvantaged areas. One way to do this is to enforce federal policies prohibiting discrimination in health service delivery.

Statement:

23. Federal policies prohibiting discrimination in health service delivery should be enforced.

Comment:

They should be enforced to better equate services offered.

Next, they believe that all Americans have a right—not a privilege—to health care.

Statement:

21. I believe that *all* Americans have a right—not a privilege—to health care.

Comment:

Think about it. We have a "right" to bear arms—a means by which life might be taken—why not the opposite—preserve life through health care.

Because everyone should be able to take advantage of technology, health. You shouldn't have to earn good health.

This is coupled with their belief that to reach minority populations effectively with prevention information requires messages and programs tailored for a specific audience and that people are more likely to participate when they are recognized as a person rather than labeled into minority groups.

They agree that any successful health campaign should originate at the community, rather than state or national, level. However, they do not necessarily think it is important to enlist the help of community leaders. They seem to have more faith in government's ability to fix the health care system than other subjects do.

This group tends to focus on economic barriers, but dismisses other types of barriers. For example, The Fixers believe rich people are better able to obtain quality medical care.

Statement:

42. Rich people get better medical care than poor people.

Comment:

Routine care is too expensive for the average American.

However, they don't think transportation is a barrier to health care, they don't think doctors are prejudiced against blacks, and they doubt that African Americans are reluctant to obtain early treatment for illnesses because care is provided by white medical personnel. They disagree with the notion that the federal government's health policies are geared for the general population and do not help minorities very much. They do think there is a health care crisis in this country, possibly because care is not up to the standard they think is obtainable. However, they are optimistic that a health care system that gives everyone the help they need is possible.

Statement:

5.   We don't have a health care crisis in this country.

Comment:

It is obvious there is a health care crisis in this country.

We do have a crisis when the wealthiest industrialized western civilization has the poorest health care.

Although they do not care whether their own physicians are black or white, they do think that physicians and health care practitioners need to respect the pride, values, and folkways of people they are trying to reach. They also are the most likely of the types to agree that one way to "fix" the system and provide adequate health care for African Americans is to educate more black health care providers.

The Fixers also are concerned about "fixing" themselves. They strongly disagree that there is not much they can do to keep from getting sick, but they acknowledge that they might not know all they need to know to stay well.

Statement:

7.   There is not much I can do to keep from getting sick.

Comment:

Prevention is a viable alternative—and an imperative one.

Statement:

34. I know all I need to know about how to stay well.

Comment:

I don't know enough about anything.

The Fixers agree that the ability of a doctor to help them depends in large part on their belief that the doctor will help them. They believe in concern for the future as well as today.

Statement:

6.   The future will take care of itself; I only need to worry about today.

Comment:

The future is dictated by today.

The future takes care of itself, but I need to take care of my future—if I can.

The idea that God might use illness as a punishment appears to stem from the belief that there might be something wrong in their lives that God is warning them to make right.

Statement:

17.   Illness can be a punishment from God.

Comment:

God do [sic] bring us down sometimes and illness could be his technique.

They are less likely to believe that the real key to good health is to lead a clean, moral life. They do find the time to go to the doctor if they are not feeling well, and they don't think getting the care they need is too much trouble. They are the least likely to go to an emergency room for routine medical care.

Statement:

16.   If I need medical care, I will most likely go to a hospital emergency room rather than to a private physician.

Comment:

I would go to a primary care doctor, lower costs, etc.

The Fixers think that the lack of access to basic health care is an urgent issue troubling American society. They expect that people suspected of not having insurance will have longer waits at hospitals. Interestingly, they believe it is not more important for an American health care system to give free medical care to the poor than to the middle or upper income person, possibly because they think it is equally important for all groups.

The Fixers are the least likely to think television is the best vehicle for important health messages, but they still consider television more appropriate than newspapers. This is possibly because they personally do not take the time to read newspaper and magazine health articles. All read newspapers, and three of the four read a black newspaper. However, only one regularly reads newspaper and magazine health articles. The others read them occasionally. Two said they generally believe the articles they read, one usually questions them, and one said it depends on the source.

Although this is a small group, its members are the healthiest of all the types. They do see a health care system in crisis, but they do not blame racism or transportation barriers for the problems. Rather, they are concerned with economic barriers. In spite of their tendency to be fixers, they are not looking to the government to solve the problems because they seem to think government programs are not helping minorities. They are much more likely to prefer individual or community-based efforts. They want to take care of themselves and would probably encourage others to do likewise.

COMPARISONS OF Q TYPES

Z-scores indicate whether the types rank statements positively or negatively. The statements that are uniquely ranked by each type are discussed below according to whether they ranked the statements greater or less than other types. (Note: This does not necessarily mean that they ranked them in opposition to other types. For example, all types might rank a statement positively, but one type ranks it more positively than the others.)

The Equalizers rank only six statements greater than the other types. They are the most concerned about transportation to health care facilities. They believe it is appropriate to use newspapers to disperse health care information. They see lack of access as an urgent issue, and they want the health system to be overhauled. They do not believe federal policies help minorities. They disagree to a lesser extent than other types that blacks are reluctant to be served by white health care practitioners. There are several statements that they rank less than the other types. They believe there is a health care crisis. Racial barriers are an issue to them, and they may care more than other types about the race of their doctors. The Equalizers disagree that a successful health care campaign should originate in the community. They don't believe they only have to worry about today, and they will not go to a doctor only if they believe they are sick. They do not avoid doctors out of fear, and they discuss illnesses in their families.

The Adjusters rank five statements greater than the other types. They agree that access to health care is out of the reach of those not able to pay. They agree that blacks are victims of the economic system, that rich people getter better care than poor people, that minorities have not been taught to use the system, and that all Americans have a right to health care. They rank seven statements less than the others. They do not believe that messages should be labeled as black health care concerns, that there is not much they can do to keep from getting sick, that African Americans avoid the system because of white practitioners, or that people are more likely to participate when they are recognized as persons rather than part of a minority group. They believe that churches do have a role in promoting health, and they do not think illness is a punishment from God. They agree, but to a lesser extent than the other types, that they might take preventive action to save money later.

The Preventers rank several statements greater than all others. They have pride in the health care system, and they have no trouble finding time to go to the doctor. Members of this type believe there is a health care crisis in the country. They believe the key to good health is to lead a clean, moral life, and they do not know enough about staying well. They do read health care articles, but they believe important health care messages should be put on television. This type believes that support groups are important and that community leaders are important to the success of a health campaign. The Preventers rank fourteen statements less than the other types. These include statements about enforcing federal policies against discrimination, disagreement that doctors are prejudiced, disagreement that the health care system makes them feel poor, and belief that Americans have a right rather than a privilege to health care. They disagree that the whole health care system should be overhauled. Most of the other statements they rank less have to do with barriers and racial prejudice. The Preventers do not acknowledge, to the same magnitude as other types, that barriers exist.

The Empathizers rank statements greater than other types that have to do with media bias and economic barriers. For example, they believe the media are prejudiced, that it is more important to give free medical care to the poor than to middle and upper income people, and that lacking insurance means long waits for medical service. They also may avoid doctors, or at least think that faith in their doctors in necessary before physicians can help them. They are the least likely to go to an emergency room. Members of this type do not find racial barriers in the health care system. They especially do not care whether their health care providers are black or white.

The Fixers rank statements greater than other types that concern improving preventive efforts in disadvantaged areas, providing more black health care providers, acknowledging that not everyone has equal access to health care, and acknowledging that the health care system makes them feel poor. They prefer messages tailored for specific audiences and believe that successful campaigns should originate at the community level. The statements they rank less than other types involve knowing all they need to know about staying well, giving free care to the poor, having no trouble going to the doctor, and using television to disperse important health messages. They are not concerned about reading health care articles or obtaining transportation to their doctor's office. They also disagree that federal policies benefit minorities.

CONCLUSIONS

Subjects seem to reflect expected trends in line with the media research and health care research cited previously in this book except for use of hospital emergency rooms. Since there are adequate statistics to indicate large segments of the African American population use emergency rooms rather than going to private doctors for illnesses that could be handled by a general practitioner or clinic, there is concern that this part of the population is not adequately represented in this phase of the study. The telephone survey that concludes this study also will be important in determining whether segments of the population may be under-represented.

Perhaps the most unexpected finding is an attitude toward the importance of black health care workers and physicians. The African American subjects strongly believe that it does not matter whether their physicians are black or white as long as their needs are being met. The predominantly black types also do not accept the idea that training more black health care practitioners and doctors would solve health care system problems.

Although there are no statements that directly relate to attitudes about family physicians, whites in the sample are more likely to have a family physician than are the African Americans, even though the African Americans are more likely to have a seen a doctor in the past year. Contrary to established statistics about the use of the emergency room, there did not seem to be any more reliance on the emergency room among the African Americans than among the whites.

Attitudinally, both blacks and whites seem to think that prevention is important, but the whites in the sample have made more changes in diet and exercise habits than have African Americans. On the other hand, African Americans have reduced tobacco and alcohol consumption.

In terms of the original hypotheses, some preliminary observations are possible. As the previous discussion illustrates, the target audiences can be segmented into groups (Q types) that have distinct attitude patterns. The attitude pattern for one type has been compared and contrasted with all other types. H1 is, therefore, confirmed.

There is much evidence that there are variations of attitude toward health care within the African American audience. African Americans are found on all Q types which indicates that there is not one uniform attitude pattern for all black Americans. H2 is confirmed.

As a group, African Americans seem to be more dependent on the media. At least they spend more hours on the average watching television and listening to the radio compared to the Caucasians in the sample. But, they are less exposed to newspapers and reported less interest in health articles in general. There also are variations in media exposure among the Q types. The Empathizers, for example, reported the highest amount of television viewership and radio listenership. The Preventers are not likely to be exposed to black newspapers. The Fixers seem to be the least interested in reading health articles in newspapers and magazines. Because different media exposure and reliance patterns are evident, H3 is confirmed.

By and large physicians are the No. 1 source of health information for those participating in the Q sort. However, both The Adjusters and The Fixers are not as dependent on doctors for information as the other Q types. They do appear to be more media dependent that the others. Despite focus group suggestions that family members had not passed along information about the genetic transmission of diabetes susceptibility, African Americans in this study deny that they do not discuss illnesses in their families. They also ranked family and friends as sources of health information higher than did those in the white population. As stated, H4 is not supported because media sources are not more influential for the majority and because reliance on either media sources or interpersonal sources may vary across Q types.

Although there are variations among the factors, the predominately black types seem to agree that there are economic, transportation, and racial barriers to receiving health care, while the predominately white types focus more on just the economic barriers. The only Q type (The Preventers) that agrees that it has pride in the American health care system is predominantly white. H5 is confirmed.

Perhaps the most important conclusion to be reached here is that there are distinctly unique attitudes held by some African Americans and some unique attitudes held by some whites. The most striking area of difference is that the predominately black type has no pride in the American health care system, but the predominately white type does have pride in the system. The largest type cuts across racial lines, but there is some evidence that this can be an economic effect. Middle class blacks and middle class whites seem more in agreement than upper income whites and low income blacks. The next chapter, which details the results of the telephone survey, will shed more light on this particular conclusion.

CHAPTER VIII

Telephone Survey Expansion of the Q Types

Following is an analysis of the clusters obtained from the telephone survey that is used to extend the Q types—The Equalizers, The Adjusters, The Preventers, The Empathizers, and The Fixers. As previously mentioned, all but one of the statements that comprised the Q sample for the previous component of this study were used for the first part of the telephone survey. Some statements were edited slightly to make administering them over the telephone easier.

When means are used to determine significance for results displayed in tabular form, an (*) indicates significance at the .05 level and an (**) indicates significance at the .01 level. Statements with means significantly below 3.0 indicate agreement, and statements with means significantly above than 3.0 indicate disagreement. Statements not significantly different from the mean indicate neutrality.

THE EQUALIZERS

The Equalizers form the largest cluster with 135 members. About 42% are from Kansas City, 39% from St. Louis, and 19% from Baton Rouge, which means that 82% are from Missouri and 19% are from Louisiana. This is a predominantly Caucasian cluster (69%).

The Equalizers' lowest mean (indicating agreement) is for the statement that shows no concern about their doctors' race (Q62). Other reactions to the statements also show that racism is not an issue with them. They are not reluctant to obtain early treatment for illnesses because care is provided mainly by white medical personnel (Q19), and they do not view African Americans as victims (Q22) or think federal health policies do not help minorities (Q59). They do not think physicians are prejudiced against

African Americans (Q21). However, they do acknowledge that there could be racial barriers to health care (Q54).

They exhibit concern that there is unequal health care in the United States, and they want treatment equalized. This can be accomplished through the enforcement of federal policies prohibiting discrimination in health service delivery (Q37) and treating all people equally and as individuals (Q33, Q35, Q50). They also see lack of access as an urgent social issue (Q38), believe the health care delivery system needs to be overhauled (Q58), and that there is a health care crisis (Q15). They lack pride in the current system (Q59).

The highest mean for this cluster (indicating disagreement) is for the statement that illness is a punishment from God (Q31). They are not fatalistic about their health (Q20, Q16) and exhibit concerned with preventing illness, both for themselves and others. Their second lowest mean is with the statement that preventive health efforts must be improved in disadvantaged areas (Q52).

They believe there are steps they can take to prevent illness (Q16, Q27), getting care is not too much trouble (Q24), and transportation is personally not a problem (Q17). They do not avoid doctors (Q57). However, they are not sure that they have all the information they need to stay well (Q45).

Members of this cluster believe that support groups are important because people relate to others like themselves (Q18), and illnesses are discussed in their families (Q47).

Regarding mass communication, The Equalizers believe that health campaigns should not be labeled as concerns only for African Americans (Q40), although they think messages should be targeted toward minority audiences (Q44). They agree that important health care messages should be put on television (Q29), but they also take time to read health stories in newspapers and magazines (Q51). They also believe churches should promote better health (Q41), and that successful campaigns should originate at the community level (Q39).

In summary, this group sees many problems with the health care system, but they do not think racism is at the heart of those problems. Although they exhibit sensitivity toward others, they take responsibility for the state of their own health. (See Table 8 for the complete means array and comparison to other clusters.)

THE ADJUSTERS

The Adjusters are the second largest cluster with 108 members. About 40% are from Kansas City, 42% from St. Louis, and 17% from Baton Rouge, which means that 82% are from Missouri, and 19% are from Louisiana (the same as The Equalizers). However, this is a predominantly African American cluster (64%).

Although the predominantly white Equalizers and predominantly black Adjusters hold many attitudes in common, The Adjusters are more urgent in their view that there are problems to solve in the American health care system. Their highest mean is for the statement that indicates there is no health care crisis in this country (Q15). Their lowest mean is for the statement that indicates preventive health efforts must be improved in disadvantaged areas (Q52). They believe that everyone has a right to health care (Q35), but not everyone has access (Q50), especially the poor (Q56).

They want health care practitioners to respect the pride, values, and folkways of the people they reach (Q33), and they think people should not be labeled or separated into minority groups.

They believe lack of access is an urgent social issue, and they want discrimination in health service delivery to be prohibited (Q37). They are more likely than The Equalizers to say that the health care system makes them feel poor (Q32) and to believe that more African American health care providers are needed (Q61). They are pessimistic that a more equitable health care system is possible (Q42).

Concerning communication methods, personal responsibility for one's health, and racism in the health care system, The Adjusters' attitudes are much like The Equalizers'. They are distinguished mostly because on of their emphasis on the poor or disadvantaged and the urgency they feel in making adjustments to the health care system. (See Table 8 for the complete means array and comparison to other clusters.)

THE PREVENTERS

The Preventers are the most geographically dispersed of the clusters. Of the 105 members, about 29% are from Kansas City, 32% from St. Louis, and 39% from Baton Rouge, which means that 61% are from Missouri and 39% are from Louisiana. As with the Q type, this is the most Caucasian cluster (73%).

Members of The Preventers cluster live up to their name in many ways. Their lowest mean is for the statement that implies they will take preventive measures now to avoid the expense of major illnesses later (Q27). They read health stories in newspapers and magazines (Q51), and they believe preventive health efforts should be improved in disadvantaged areas (Q52).

They do not care about the color of their doctors as long as they are paying attention to their needs, and they do want physicians to respect the pride, values, and folkways of their patients (Q33).

The Preventers most disagree with the statement that illnesses are not discussed in their families (Q47). The statement with the second highest mean indicates that they do not believe they only have to worry about today (Q20).

They also recognize the value of support groups (Q18) and think people will be more likely to participate when they are not labeled or separated into groups (Q48). They think health campaigns should not label diseases as concerns for only African-Americans (Q40).

They do not think that illness is a punishment from God (Q31), but they do think living a clean, moral life is important to prevent disease (Q26). They agree that the ability of a physician to help them depends on their belief that he or she can help them (Q46).

This is one of two clusters that express pride in the American health care system (Q59), and they disagree that the health care delivery system needs to be overhauled (Q58). Still, they believe federal policies prohibiting discrimination should be enforced and that everyone has a right to health care (Q35).

Originally called the *Oblivious* Preventers, this cluster dismisses or does not recognize many of the barriers to health care. They do not think African-Americans are victims of an economic system that dictates both their ability to receive health services and the quality of their health (Q22). They said the health care system does not make them feel poor (Q32) and that lacking insurance does not translate into long waits for services (Q49). They do not think minorities have been taught how to use the health care system (Q60), although they believe government policies help minorities (Q53). They do not think more black health care providers will solve problems of adequate health care for African-Americans (Q61).

Although they tend to consider both television and newspapers appropriate modes of health care communication, The Preventers consider television more important than newspapers (Q29, Q28). They do not think the media care only about diseases that affect Caucasians.

The Preventers support preventive actions, and they take much responsibility for their own health care. They are not concerned about barriers or racism that prevent adequate health care. In fact, they have faith in the current American health care system. (See Table 8 for the complete means array and comparison to other clusters.)

THE EMPATHIZERS

Of the 115 members of The Empathizers, 38% are from Kansas City, 44% are from St. Louis, and 17% are from Baton Rouge, which means that 83% are from Missouri and 17% are from Louisiana. This is a racially mixed cluster that is 44% Caucasian and 57% African-American.

In many ways, The Empathizers are the hardest to characterize. They have general tendencies for most of their viewpoints, but they do not hold extreme opinions toward any of the statements. In some cases, the cluster seems to divide in attitude along racial lines (according to crosstabulations of this cluster's responses by race).

First, they do not care whether their doctors are black or white (Q62), but they expect their physicians to respect the pride, values, and folkways of their patients (Q33). Second, they believe in the right of all Americans to receive health care (Q35), and they want preventive efforts to be improved in disadvantaged areas (Q52).

They also believe support groups are important (Q18). They will personally take preventive measure today to save money tomorrow (Q27). However, they do not think they have all the information they need to stay well (Q45).

Next, they agree that everyone does not have equal access to health care (Q50) and that access is beyond those not able to pay for it (Q43). The rich get better care than the poor (Q56). They believe it is more important for an American health care system to give free medical care to the disadvantaged than to middle and upper income citizens (Q23). Consequently, they think there is a health care crisis (Q15), that lack of access is an urgent social issue (Q38), and that the whole delivery system needs to be overhauled (Q58).

Although the statement with which they most disagree (Q17) indicates transportation is not a problem for them, The Empathizers are likely to go to a hospital emergency room rather than to a private physician (Q30). They say they will go to a doctor only if they are sick (Q55). They expect that people will have to wait for service if they do not have insurance (Q49), and they also think African-Americans are the victims of an economic system that determines whether they receive adequate health care (Q22).

The Empathizers also prefer that health campaigns do not single out African-Americans (Q48). Although they personally read health care articles in newspapers and magazines, they rate television higher than newspapers as sources for health messages (Q29, Q28). They think community leaders are important to the success of a health campaign (Q34).

Members of this cluster do not avoid doctors, and they also tend to agree that they have to believe in their doctor's ability to help them (Q46). They do not think doctors are prejudiced against their black patients (Q21).

The key to good health, in their view, is to lead a clean, moral life (Q26). They do not see illness as a punishment from God (Q31). They also believe they have to be concerned about the future (Q20). They also believe there are actions they can take to prevent illness (Q16). They discuss illnesses with family members (Q47) and do not think getting health care is too much trouble (Q24).

They are somewhat divided about racial barriers. Although they do not think the media demonstrate prejudice in coverage of health issues (Q25), they believe it is important to train more black health care providers (Q61). They are not bothered by receiving health care from white medical personnel (Q19), but they do not want discrimination in health service delivery (Q37).

The best picture of this group is that they are concerned about the economic difficulties associated with adequate health care, and they believe major changes in the system are in order. Because of the racial mixture of respondents, they tend to recognize some unfairness in the system, but they do not go so far as to blame racism for the system's problems. They do not avoid the health care system, and they are willing to accept personal responsibility for their health; but they are more likely than the other clusters to postpone treatment (possibly for economic reasons) until they are really ill. (See Table 8 for the complete means array and comparison to other clusters.)

THE FIXERS

The smallest of the clusters (and also of the Q types) is The Fixers with 63 members. Fifty percent are from Kansas City, 38% are from St. Louis, and 11% are from Baton Rouge, which means that 89% are from Missouri and 11% are from Louisiana. Eighty-three percent of this cluster is African-American.

The Fixers tend to agree with the majority of the statements. Many have a mean between 1.635 and 2.825. Only one statement, with a mean of 3.677, shows any significant degree of disagreement. The remaining 11 statements fall in the neutral area between means of 2.730 and 3.190. (See Table 8.)

The Fixers demonstrate much concern about fixing the health care system to better serve the poor and disadvantaged. The statements with means below 2 (Q56, Q35, Q52, Q33, Q37, Q43, Q50, Q62, Q61, Q49, Q38, Q48, Q26, Q58) all deal with the rich and advantaged receiving access to better health care than the poor and disadvantaged or with concerns about racial or social distinctions. They include statements about physicians respecting the culture of their patients, prohibiting discrimination, lack of concern about whether physicians are black or white, and lack of access. Additional statements deal with lack of insurance, providing more black health care providers, avoiding labeling and separating people into minority groups, and ultimately overhauling the entire health care system.

Additionally, the statement with the highest mean (Q15) indicates that The Fixers believe there is a health care crisis in this country. Still, they did express pride in the American health care system (Q59).

The statements with means between 2 and 3 involve both self control over illness and media messages. The Fixers are willing to take preventive action to save money down the line (Q27), although they tend to agree that there is not much they can do to keep from getting sick (Q16). They believe support groups are important (Q18), and they think a doctor's ability to help them depends on their belief that the doctor will help them (Q46). However, they may go to a doctor only if they think they have a health problem (Q55). They agree that both television and newspapers are important ways to transmit health care messages (Q27, Q28), but they consider television the more important source (mean of 2.000 for television, compared to 2.274 for newspapers). They believe community leaders are important to the success of a health campaign (Q34).

Also within this mean range, The Fixers agree that health campaigns should not single out African-Americans (Q40), that messages and program should be tailored for and targeted to a specific audience (Q44), that African-Americans are victims of the economic system (Q22), and that it is more important for the health care system to give free medical care to the poor and disadvantaged rather than to middle and upper income citizens (Q23). They agree that minorities have not been taught how to use the health care system (Q60). They do not think federal health policies help minorities (Q53), and they think both the media and physicians can be prejudiced against African-Americans (Q21). They also agree that blacks are more likely than other groups to die from diseases that can be cured or managed.

Members of this cluster also are likely to go to a hospital emergency room rather than to a private physician (Q30), and they indicate that the health care system makes them feel like they are poor (Q32).

This cluster is concerned with both economic and racial issues associated with health care. However, even though they want the system overhauled, they still indicate pride in the current system. They may be more fatalistic than other clusters about their health, but they also are willing to take preventive actions that are within their economic means. (See Table 8 for the complete means array and comparison to other clusters.)

CLUSTER COMPARISONS

Examining the means provides a method for comparing differences among the clusters. (See Table 8.) For example, The Fixers is the only cluster to agree that doctors are prejudiced against blacks (Q21). Members of this cluster also are the only ones to agree that there is not much they can do to keep from getting sick (Q16). They are the only ones to think that getting health care is too much trouble (Q24). Of all the clusters they agree the most that they only need to worry about today because the future will take of itself (Q20).

The Fixers cluster has the lowest mean for the statement that the real key to good health is to lead a clean, moral life (Q26). The Preventers and Empathizers also agree, while The Equalizers and The Adjusters disagree.

The Fixers have the strongest degree of agreement that lack of insurance means longer waits for treatment (Q49). (The Preventers is the only cluster to disagree with this statement.)

Both The Adjusters and The Fixers agree that the health care system makes them feel poor, but the other clusters either are neutral or disagree (Q32). These clusters also agree that federal policies do not help minorities, while The Equalizers and The Preventers disagree and The Empathizers are neutral (Q53).

Both The Equalizers and The Preventers do not see African-Americans as the victims of the economic system, while the other clusters agree with this statement (Q22). Members of these two clusters also are the only ones who said they would use a private physician rather than go to the emergency room for immediate care (Q30).

The Adjusters cluster is the only one to lack pride in the American health care system (Q59). The Adjusters and The Fixers agree that minorities have not been taught how to use the health care system (Q60). Theses clusters also agree that the media can be prejudiced against black health concerns, but the other clusters disagree (Q25). The Adjusters and The Empathizers believe that racial barriers to health care are an issue, while The Preventers believe they are not an issue. The other two groups are neutral (Q54). The Empathizers and The Fixers agree that they will go to their doctor only if they think something is wrong with their health. The other clusters are neutral (Q55). The Adjusters show the most agreement toward the knowledge statement that African-Americans are more likely to die from diseases that can be cured or managed than are other minority groups and

TABLE 8

STATISTICAL COMPARISON OF CLUSTER MEANS

Statement		Equalizers	Adjusters	Preventers	Empathizers	Fixers
Q15	We do not have a heatlh care crisis in this country.	4.304**	4.596**	3.057	3.652**	3.677**
Q16	There is not much I can do to keep from getting sick.	4.037**	4.000**	3.848**	3.342*	2.317**
Q17	I can't get heatlh care because I have no transportation to and from a doctor's office, clinic, or hospital.	4.059**	4.019**	4.067**	3.739**	3.159
Q18	Support groups are important because many people can relate to others who are like themselves.	1.778**	1.789**	1.981**	2.139**	2.016**
Q19	I am reluctant to obtain early treatment for illnesses because care is provided mainly by white medical personnel.	4.207**	4.065**	4.067**	3.617**	3.111
Q20	I only need to worry about today because the future will take care of itself.	4.326**	4.275**	4.095**	3.652**	2.730
Q21	Many doctors are prejudiced against African-Americans.	3.537**	3.156	3.819**	3.217*	2.683*
Q22	African-Americans are the victims of an economic system that dictates both their ability to receive health services and the quality of their health.	3.200*	1.826**	3.971**	2.783*	2.190**

TABLE 8 *(continued)*

Statement		Equalizers	Adjusters	Preventers	Empathizers	Fixers
Q23	It is more important for an American health care system to give free medical care to the poor and disadvantaged than to give free care to middle and upper income citizens.	2.748*	2.444**	2.905	2.623**	2.222**
Q24	Getting the heath care I need is usually too much trouble.	4.000**	3.670**	3.933**	3.409**	2.810
Q25	As long as a disease is hitting white people, the media care. But if it's hitting mainly African Americans, they are not going to worry about it too much.	3.526**	1.963**	3.962**	3.377**	2.677*
Q26	The real key to good health is to lead a clean, moral life.	3.037	3.229	2.524**	2.389**	1.952**
Q27	If I can save money down the line, I might take preventive measures now to avoid the expense of having a heart attack and paying doctors bills or whatever.	1.741**	1.826**	1.769**	2.200**	2.000**
Q28	It is appropriate to use newspapers to try to get information out about health risks such heart disease and diabetes.	1.993**	2.101**	2.514**	2.626**	2.274**
Q29	If you have an important message about health care, put it on television.	2.007**	2.028**	2.162**	2.409**	2.000**

TABLE 8 *(continued)*

Statement	Equalizers	Adjusters	Preventers	Empathizers	Fixers
Q30 If I need immediate medical care, I probably would go to a hospital emergency room rather than to a private physician.	3.126	2.771*	3.152	2.287**	2.333**
Q31 Illness can be a punishment from God	4.415**	4.296**	3.943**	3.635**	3.000
Q32 The heatlh care system makes me feel like I'm poor.	3.178	2.716*	3.876**	3.096	2.355**
Q33 Physicians and heatlh care practitioners need to respect the pride, values, and folkways of people they are trying to reach.	1.748**	1.523**	2.048**	2.105**	1.810**
Q34 Community leaders (such as teachers and preachers) are important to the success of any heatlh care campaign.	2.104**	2.110**	2.400**	2.522**	2.143**
Q35 I believe that all Americans have a right—not a privilege—to health care.	1.793**	1.505**	2.533**	2.078**	1.651**
Q36 If I'm not feeling well, I have no trouble finding time to go to the doctor.	2.667*	2.780	2.810	2.896	2.524**
Q37 Federal policies prohibiting discrimination in health service delivery should be enforced.	1.785**	1.615**	2.279**	2.389**	1.823**
Q38 Lack of access to basic heatlh care is an urgent social issue.	1.859**	1.624**	3.190	2.482**	1.921**
Q39 Any successful health campaign that could change behaviors would have to originate in my community, not at the state or national level.	3.276*	2.899	2.657*	2.885	2.452**

TABLE 8 (continued)

Statement		Equalizers	Adjusters	Preventers	Empathizers	Fixers
Q40	Health campaigns for particular diseases should emphasize that these are health care concerns for all people, rather than labeling them as just concerns for African Americans.	1.859**	1.716**	2.143**	2.342**	2.032**
Q41	Churches really have no role in promoting better physical health.	3.348**	3.725**	3.524**	3.281*	2.825
Q42	A heatlh care system that gives everyone the help they need is never going to happen.	3.141	2.963	3.029	2.851	2.790
Q43	Access to heatlh care and to the means of maintaining health are simply out of the reach of those not able to pay.	2.615**	1.890**	3.695**	2.272**	1.825**
Q44	To reach minorities effectively with prevention information requires messages and programs that are tailored for and targeted to reach a specific audience.	2.082**	1.936**	2.648**	2.717*	2.063**
Q45	I know all I need to know about how to stay well.	3.689**	3.752**	3.486**	3.504**	2.762
Q46	The ability of a doctor to help me depends in large part on my belief that the doctor will help me.	2.289**	2.275**	2.324**	2.383**	2.063**
Q47	Illnesses are not discussed in my family.	4.311**	4.055**	4.114**	3.687**	3.190

TABLE 8 *(continued)*

Statement		Equalizers	Adjusters	Preventers	Empathizers	Fixers
Q48	People are more likely to participate when they are recognized as a person, rather than being labeled, isolated and separated into minority groups.	1.748**	1.569**	2.057**	2.219**	1.937**
Q49	If you go to a hospital and they figure you may not have insurance or you're undercovered, they always make you wait. But, if you have insurance, they take you right in.	3.075	2.174**	3.519**	2.675**	1.903**
Q50	Everyone does not have equal access to health care.	1.911**	1.550**	2.952	2.202**	1.841**
Q51	I take the time to read health stories in newspapers and magazines.	2.007**	2.055**	2.067**	2.365**	2.333**
Q52	Preventive health efforts must be improved in disadvantaged areas.	1.719**	1.477**	2.125**	2.174**	1.683**
Q53	The federal government's health policies are geared for the general population. They don't help minorities very much.	3.373**	2.642*	3.752**	3.053	2.476**
Q54	Racial barriers to health care are not an issue.	3.410**	3.862**	2.788*	3.035	2.774
Q55	I will go to a doctor only if I think something is wrong with my health.	3.156	3.037	3.000	2.565**	2.222**
Q56	Rich people get better medical care than poor people.	1.881**	1.550**	2.629**	2.330**	1.635**

TABLE 8 *(continued)*

Statement		Equalizers	Adjusters	Preventers	Empathizers	Fixers
Q57	My inclination is to stay away from doctors because you're not really sick until the doctor says you are.	4.157**	4.028**	4.057**	3.704**	3.111
Q58	The whole heatlh care delivery system needs to be overhauled.	1.933**	1.734**	3.562**	2.209**	1.984**
Q59	I have a great deal of pride in the American heatlh care system.	3.363**	3.495**	2.171**	2.974	2.127**
Q60	Minorities have not been taught how to use the health care system.	3.096	1.954**	3.533**	3.053	2.286**
Q61	The ultimate solution to providing adequate health care for African Americans is to educate enough black heatlh care providers to do it.	3.000	2.734*	3.279*	2.739**	1.889**
Q62	It doesn't matter to me whether doctors are black or white as long as they pay attention to my needs.	1.548**	1.761**	1.857**	2.009**	1.857**
Q63	Blacks are more likely to die from diseases that can be cured or managed than are other minority groups and whites.	2.726*	1.972**	3.105	2.939	2.349**

whites (1.972). Both the Preventers and The Empathizers are neutral toward the knowledge question.

Members of The Preventers cluster are the only ones to disagree that the health care system needs to be overhauled (Q58). This is the only cluster that does not think access to health care is out of the reach of those not able to pay (Q43). They also are the only ones to disagree that the ultimate solution to providing adequate health care for African-Americans is to educate enough black health care providers (Q61).

MEDIA USE, DEMOGRAPHIC COMPARISONS

Once the audience has been successfully segmented, (thus far by factor and cluster), the next step is to examine media habits, health status, and general demographics by cluster. Once this is accomplished, specific strategies concerning message content and dispersion can be planned. The following sections compare the clusters in terms of media reliance, general health and lifestyle, and along standard demographics. These comparisons rely on crosstabulation tables and Chi-Square tests of statistical significance at the .05 level.

MEDIA USE

As the following table shows, there are differences in the average number of hours members of each cluster spend watching television and listening to the radio each week.

TABLE 9
TELEVISION/RADIO HOURS PER WEEK

Cluster	Television Hours /Week	Radio Hours/Week
The Equalizers	16.4 N=133	13.4 N=134
The Preventers	19.3 N=104	14.5 N=104
The Empathizers	21 N=112	15.8 N=114
The Adjusters	15.7 N=108	12.8 N=109
The Fixers	26 N=63	23.3 N=62

The Adjusters and The Equalizers have the lowest average weekly hours of television viewing, while The Fixers have the highest average viewing. The Fixers watch television the greatest average number of hours, while The Adjusters listen the least number on average.

As would be expected, the clusters containing the largest African-American populations have the highest percentage of black radio station listeners. Sixty percent of The Fixers, 57% of The Adjusters, 43% of The Empathizers, 26% of the Equalizers, and 20% of The Preventers listen to a black radio station (p=.00000).

There are major differences in regular newspaper readership. Seventy-five percent of The Adjusters, 74% of The Preventers, 73% of The Equalizers, 64% of The Empathizers, and 54% of The Fixers subscribe to or regularly read newspapers. Fifty percent of The Adjusters, 41% of The Fixers, 33% of The Empathizers, 25% of The Equalizers, and 13% of The Preventers, read black newspapers (p=.00001).

SOURCES OF HEALTH CARE INFORMATION

Although there are no statistically significant differences in interpersonal sources among the clusters, there are differences in media sources. Physicians are clearly the major source for every cluster.

TABLE 10
INTERPERSONAL SOURCES

Sources	Percentage in Each Cluster				
	Equalizers	Preventers	Empathizers	Adjusters	Fixers
Doctors	57%	63%	55%	48%	61%
Nurses	6%	6%	4%	6%	2%
Family members	15%	10%	13%	19%	19%
Friends	5%	6%	12%	12%	5%
Multiple sources	8%	11%	7%	7%	7%
No sources	9%	6%	9%	8%	7%
N=523	135	105	112	109	62

The Fixers are the most dependent on television (56%), and The Empathizers are the least likely to have a source (6%). However, most clusters rely on a variety of sources (p=.02186).

TABLE 11
MEDIA SOURCES

Sources	Percentage in Each Cluster				
	Equalizers	Preventers	Empathizers	Adjusters	Fixers
Newspapers	20%	21%	14%	24%	12%
Magazines	28%	17%	14%	26%	15%
Radio	3%	5%	8%	7%	7%
Television	28%	31%	33%	30%	46%
Medical publications	18%	24%	25%	10%	18%
Multiple sources	1%	2%	0%	0%	2%
No sources	2%	1%	6%	3%	2%
N=514	134	105	107	107	61

READERSHIP OF HEALTH ARTICLES

The Equalizers are the most likely to regularly (59%) or occasionally (36%) read health articles in newspapers and magazines. Both The Fixers and The Empathizers are the least likely to read them. Almost 29% of The Fixers and 23% of The Empathizers said they rarely or never read these types of articles (p=.00001).

The readership for each type of article by group follows:

TABLE 12
HEALTH ARTICLE READERSHIP BY CLUSTERS

Article Type	Percentage of Readers by Cluster				
	Equalizers	Preventers	Empathizers	Adjusters	Fixers
Diet & Nutrition N=526 (p=.00008)	88%	88%	77%	90%	66%
Exercise N=525 (p=.03106)	84%	87%	73%	83%	73%
Diabetes N=526 (p=.01714)	74%	67%	68%	82%	60%
Heart/ High **Blood Pressure** N=526 (p=.29934)	87%	88%	80%	89%	82%

TABLE 12 *(continued)*

Article Type	Percentage of Readers by Cluster				
	Equalizers	Preventers	Empathizers	Adjusters	Fixers
Glaucoma/ Eye Disease N=527 (p=.02033)	56%	65%	50%	71%	60%
Sickle Cell Anemia N=525 (p=.00028)	42%	43%	47%	68%	56%
Cancer N=526 (p=.01754)	91%	88%	78%	89%	79%
Elderly Diseases N=526 (p=.08034)	71%	71%	65%	76%	57%
Child/Infant Health N=525 (p=.35110)	62%	53%	55%	65%	60%
Stress N=526 (p=.00098)	89%	84%	73%	92%	79%
AIDS N=526 (p=.00001)	87%	66%	70%	90%	76%
General Health N=525 (p=.02462)	92%	91%	80%	92%	89%

Some cluster members are more questioning than others of the health information they read (p=.05192). The Equalizers are the most likely to believe the health articles they read (50% said they generally believe them), while The Adjusters are the most likely to question this type of information (48%). The Fixers are the most likely to consider the source (31%).

TABLE 13
HEALTH ARTICLE BELIEVABILITY

Level	Percentage in Each Cluster				
	Equalizers	Preventers	Empathizers	Adjusters	Fixers
Generally believes	50%	40%	36%	32%	42%
Usually questions	31%	37%	39%	48%	27%
Depends on source	19%	23%	25%	20%	31%
N=514	135	105	112	109	59

HEALTH STATUS

About the same percentage of each cluster are smokers (between 21% and 28%), and about the same percentage of each cluster have quit smoking within the past two years (between 5% and 9%). About the same percentage of each cluster currently drinks alcoholic beverages at least once a week (between 15% and 28%) or has quit or reduced the intake amount (10% to 12%). There are no statistically significant differences among the clusters.

However, some clusters are more likely to have taken action to improve either their own or their family's health in the past year (p=.00285). The Equalizers are the most likely to have taken action (94%) and The Fixers are the least likely to have taken action (77%). It is important to note, however, that substantial percentages in each cluster have already made changes in behavior that affects their health.

TABLE 14
LIFESTYLE CHANGES BY CLUSTERS

Change	Percentage of Change by Cluster				
	Equalizers	Preventers	Empathizers	Adjusters	Fixers
Modified diet N=492 (p=.03293)	86%	85%	75%	84%	69%
Increased exercise N=519 (p=.16371)	68%	55%	55%	64%	56%
Reduced stress N=514 (p=.31215)	69%	58%	64%	70%	60%

There also are some differences in the type of chronic illnesses prevalent in each cluster.

TABLE 15
CHRONIC DISEASE BY CLUSTERS

Disease	Percentage in Each Cluster				
	Equalizers	Preventers	Empathizers	Adjusters	Fixers
Diabetes N=518 (p=.06213)	4%	14%	12%	8%	8%
Glaucoma/ Eye Disease N=518 (p=.05167)	3%	9%	6%	4%	13%
High Blood Pressure N=520 (p=.00150)	20%	28%	27%	19%	45%
Heart/Coronary Artery Disease N=521 (p=.69339)	7%	10%	9%	8%	13%
High Cholesterol N=508 (p=.30453)	17%	22%	11%	20%	16%
Lung/Respiratory Disease N=521 (p=.22377)	8%	5%	9%	14%	8%
Cancer N=521 (p=.24134)	5%	3%	5%	3%	10%
Stroke/Brain Impairment N=524 (p=.47354)	2%	3%	2%	0%	3%
Arthritis N=516 (p=.80176)	25%	26%	26%	20%	27%

There are no statistically significant differences among the clusters in terms of whether members had seen a physician in the past year. The percentages ranged from 84% for The Empathizers to 90% for The Equalizers. Between 13% and 21% of each cluster has been hospitalized in the past year. Between 21% and 33% of each cluster has a family members who has been hospitalized in the past year.

There are significant differences among the clusters in terms of having a family physician. Seventy-six percent of The Fixers, 81% of The Empathizers, 89% of The Adjusters, 91% of The Preventers, and 93% of The Equalizers have family physicians (p=.00382).

MEDICARE, MEDICAID, INSURANCE

There are differences among the clusters in regard to Medicare and Medicaid (p=.00000). The Fixers are the most likely to use Medicare (40%) or Medicaid (32%), and The Adjusters are the least likely to use Medicare (10%) or Medicaid (7%).

There also are significance differences in insurance coverage among the clusters (p=.00000). The Fixers are the least likely to have either private or group health insurance (52%), and both The Equalizers and The Preventers are the most likely to have insurance (89%).

CLINTON HEALTH PLAN

There are major differences among the clusters in terms of knowledge of and support for Pres. Clinton's health care plan (p=.00000).

TABLE 16
KNOWLEDGE OF CLINTON PLAN BY CLUSTERS

Knowledge	Percentage in Each Cluster				
	Equalizers	Preventers	Empathizers	Adjusters	Fixers
Knowledgeable	5%	22%	4%	10%	7%
Knows something	52%	45%	43%	53%	34%
Limited knowledge	40%	21%	27%	32%	26%
Knows nothing	3%	12%	26%	5%	33%
N=524	135	104	115	109	61

The Adjusters are the most likely to favor Pres. Clinton's plan to provide universal insurance coverage, while The Preventers are the most likely to oppose it (p=.00000).

TABLE 17
SUPPORT FOR CLINTON'S PLAN BY CLUSTERS

Support	Percentage in Each Cluster				
	Equalizers	Preventers	Empathizers	Adjusters	Fixers
Favors	73%	31%	59%	84%	73%
Opposes	15%	54%	19%	6%	15%
Undecided	12%	14%	22%	11%	12%
N=524	135	105	115	109	60

DEMOGRAPHICS

The Fixers have the highest percentage of subjects who have an eighth grade education or less (13%), who attended but did not graduate from high school (16%) and who have only a high school education (48%). The majority of The Empathizers are either high school graduates (30%) or have obtained some college credit (37%). The other groups have high percentages of persons who attended college, graduated from college or have advanced degrees (p=.00000).

TABLE 18
EDUCATION LEVELS

Levels	Percentage in Each Cluster				
	Equalizers	Preventers	Empathizers	Adjusters	Fixers
-8th	1%	0%	4%	1%	13%
Attended H.S.	1%	7%	13%	3%	16%
H.S. Graduate	22%	28%	30%	17%	48%
Some College	29%	25%	37%	32%	14%
Technical School	3%	5%	4%	4%	2%
College graduate	28%	17%	10%	30%	6%
Advanced	16%	19%	2%	14%	2%
N=526	135	105	115	108	63

There are also significant differences among the age groups in the clusters (p=.00879). One-third of The Fixers are 65 or older, while most of The Adjusters are between 25 and 54. The other groups have rather diverse age spans.

TABLE 19
AGE RANGES

Ranges	Percentage in Each Cluster				
	Equalizers	Preventers	Empathizers	Adjusters	Fixers
18-24	10%	13%	17%	11%	13%
25-34	23%	14%	19%	22%	21%
35-44	22%	22%	17%	31%	16%
45-54	16%	15%	11%	22%	11%
55-64	9%	15%	11%	8%	6%
65+	19%	21%	25%	7%	33%
N=521	134	104	114	106	63

The Fixers are the most likely to be single (43%) while The Preventers are the most likely to be married (64%). Both The Fixers and The Empathizers have 12% who are widowed, and both The Empathizers and The Adjusters have about 20% who are divorced or separated (p=.00003).

TABLE 20
MARITAL STATUS

Status	Percentage in Each Cluster				
	Equalizers	Preventers	Empathizers	Adjusters	Fixers
Single	33%	21%	37%	38%	43%
Married	47%	64%	31%	36%	27%
Widowed	9%	9%	12%	6%	13%
Divorced	11%	7%	20%	21%	18%
N=523	135	105	113	107	63

There are no statistically significant differences in terms of the percentage of health care workers in the clusters. The percentages of health care workers ranged from 5% of The Fixers to 16% of The Adjusters.

A high percentage of both The Fixers and The Preventers are either retired or homemakers. About one-third of The Empathizers are blue collar workers, and an additional 30% are retired. The Equalizers tend to be white collar workers, professionals, or administrators. The Adjusters can be found in every profession.

TABLE 21
OCCUPATION CATEGORIES

Categories	Percentage in Each Cluster				
	Equalizers	Preventers	Empathizers	Adjusters	Fixers
White collar	13%	12%	7%	10%	2%
Professional	16%	16%	2%	14%	10%
Technical/Support	15%	4%	15%	19%	4%
Sales	4%	5%	0%	4%	2%
Administrative	5%	1%	1%	2%	2%
Blue Collar	12%	13%	33%	21%	28%
Journalist	2%	2%	1%	1%	0%
Homemaker	7%	7%	5%	8%	2%
Student	7%	7%	5%	8%	2%
Retired	20%	28%	30%	13%	33%
N=442	117	92	92	90	51

There are variations, but no statistically significant differences in the number of persons in the household among the clusters.

TABLE 22
HOUSEHOLD SIZE

No. in Household	Percentage in Each Cluster				
	Equalizers	Preventers	Empathizers	Adjusters	Fixers
1 person	30%	16%	29%	18%	22%
2 persons	28%	39%	22%	29%	35%
3 persons	16%	21%	23%	26%	14%
4 persons	11%	13%	17%	15%	10%
5+ persons	15%	11%	9%	13%	19%
Average Number:	2.7	2.7	2.6	2.9	2.9
N=523	134	105	113	108	63

There are significant differences in yearly total household income among the clusters (p=.00000).

TABLE 23
HOUSEHOLD INCOME

Level	Percentage in Each Cluster				
	Equalizers	Preventers	Empathizers	Adjusters	Fixers
-$10,000	7%	10%	27%	10%	49%
$11,000-$19,999	18%	8%	22%	22%	27%
$20,000-$25,999	14%	12%	19%	11%	9%
$26,000-$35,999	15%	19%	12%	26%	9%
$36,000-$45,999	12%	15%	4%	11%	4%
$46,000-$55,999	14%	15%	4%	7%	2%
$56,000-$75,999	10%	7%	8%	2%	1%
$76,000-$100,000	6%	8%	2%	4%	0%
$101,000 or more	3%	6%	1%	4%	0%
N=478	125	95	99	104	55

There are significant differences in the gender divisions among the clusters (p=.00755).

TABLE 24
GENDER

Gender	Percentage in Each Cluster				
	Equalizers	Preventers	Empathizers	Adjusters	Fixers
Males	24%	39%	43%	32%	46%
Females	76%	61%	57%	68%	54%
N=527	135	105	115	109	
	63				

CHAPTER IX

African American/ Caucasian Comparisons: Telephone Survey Responses

If Q factors and clusters are ways to differentiate various segments in Grunig's innermost nest in the social marketing model, then comparing responses from African Americans and Caucasians is an approach to examine the next nest, publics. At this level, the social marketer is attempting to segment the mass audience into groups with distinct communication and behavior patterns. As was expected from the outset of this study, there are statistically significant differences between the races in both attitudes and demographics.

Responses from those subjects who identified themselves as African American or black are compared to those who identified themselves as Caucasian or white in the telephone survey. Of the total 527 subjects, 257 persons (49%) identified themselves as black or African American and 270 persons (51%) identified themselves as Caucasian or white. About 77% of the Caucasians reside in Missouri, and 23% reside in Louisiana. Eighty percent of the African Americans reside in Missouri, and 20% reside in Louisiana.

RESULTS

As this study presupposes, there are several views of the American health care system that are more likely to be held by African Americans than by Caucasians. Most of them are linked directly to racial issues. First, the African American responses to the Q sort statements used in the telephone survey will be discussed.

AFRICAN AMERICAN RESPONSES

The African Americans in this study most agree with the statement that all Americans have a right—not a privilege—to health care (Q35). (See Table 25.) Their next lowest mean scores indicate that they do not care about the race of their doctors as long as they pay attention to their needs (Q62) and that preventive health efforts must be improved in disadvantaged areas (Q52).

Others statements with means below 2 indicate that physicians need to respect the background of their patients (Q33), that people are more likely to participate when they are not separated into minority groups (Q48), that discrimination in health service delivery should be prohibited (Q37), that support groups are important (Q18), and that they might take preventive action to save health care costs later (Q27).

Statements with means between 2 and 2.5 indicate concern for lack of access to health care (Q50, Q38) and for economic disparities that result in better care for the rich (Q56, Q43, Q22, Q49). They also believe the whole health care delivery system should be overhauled (Q58). In terms of dispersing health care messages, the African Americans responding most often agree that important messages should be on television (Q29). They also read health stories in newspapers and magazines (Q51) and agree that newspapers are appropriate vehicles for health care information (Q28).

The African Americans also agree that the ability of a doctor to help them depends on their belief that he or she can help them (Q46). There is a general sense that they only need to worry about today (Q20), and that blacks are more likely than whites to die from curable or treatable diseases (Q63)

In terms of health campaigns, they believe community leaders are important (Q34) and that to reach minorities, messages and programs should be tailored for a specific audience (Q44). They also believe churches have a role in promoting health (Q41).

The statement with which the African Americans responding most disagree (mean = 3.996) is that there is not a health care crisis in American (Q15). They also disagree that they are inclined to avoid doctors (Q57), and that illnesses are not discussed in their families (Q47). Other statements with means above 3 indicate that African Americans do not believe illness is a punishment from God (Q57), that they do not lack transportation to health care facilities (Q17), and that they are not reluctant to obtain early treatment for illnesses because care is provided by white medical personnel (Q19). They do not think getting health care is too much trouble (Q24) or that they have enough information about how to stay well (Q45). They disagree that there is not much they can do to keep from getting sick (Q16).

Although they do not believe many doctors are prejudiced against African Americans (Q21), they think racial barriers to health care are an issue (Q54).

CAUCASIAN RESPONSES

The Caucasians in the telephone sample most strongly agree that they do not care whether their doctors are black or white (Q62). (See Table 25.) Next, they agree that they might take preventive action to save medical expenses later (Q27), and that physicians need to respect their patients' pride and background (Q33).

The Caucasians, like the African Americans, agree that preventive health efforts must be improved in disadvantaged areas (Q52) and that people should not be labeled or separated into minority groups (Q48). They also think support groups are important (Q18).

The statements with means between 2 and 2.87 show concern for an equitable health care system. First, the Caucasians in the sample believe that health campaigns should not label concerns for only African Americans (Q40). Next, they believe that rich people get better medical care than poor people (Q56), that federal policies prohibiting discrimination should be enforced (Q37), and that all Americans have a right to health care (Q35). They do not believe that everyone has equal access (Q50), and they think that lack of access to basic health care is an urgent social issue (Q38).

The media statements are grouped together with means between 2.130 and 2.138. The Caucasians said they take time to reach health stories in newspapers and magazines (Q51). They equally agree that newspapers and television are appropriate vehicles for health care messages (Q28, Q29).

They also agree that community leaders are important to the success of any health care campaign and that to reach minorities, messages and programs should be tailored for a specific audience (Q44).

The Caucasians also agree with the African Americans that the health care delivery system needs to be overhauled (Q58), and that access to health care is out of the reach or those not able to pay (Q43). They also think it is more important for the poor than the middle and upper class to receive free medical care (Q23). They are pessimistic that a health care system that helps everyone is possible (Q42).

Although they said they have no trouble finding time to go to the doctor, they will go only if they think something is wrong with their health (Q55), and they think the ability of a doctor to help them depends on their faith in the doctor (Q46). They also believe the real key to good health is to lead a clean, moral life (Q26).

They also agree that blacks are more likely to die from disease that can be cured or managed than are other minority groups and whites.

The Caucasians are neutral toward eight statements, although the African Americans were neutral toward only four.

The Caucasians most strongly disagree that illness can be a punishment from God (Q31). They also strongly disagree that they only need to worry about today (Q20), that illnesses are not discussed in their families (Q47), and that they are reluctant to obtain early treatment because white personnel provide the care (Q19).

Although they do think there is a health care crisis (Q15), they are not concerned about transportation (Q17), and they do not avoid doctors (Q57). They disagree that they cannot prevent illness (Q16), and they do not think getting health care is too much trouble (Q24). However, they are not sure they have enough health information (Q24). They do not view African Americans as victims of the economic system (Q22).

They do not think either the media or physicians are prejudiced against African Americans (Q25, Q21). They disagree that federal health policies do not help minorities very much (Q53).

The Caucasians believe churches should promote better health (Q31).

AFRICAN AMERICAN/CAUCASIAN COMPARISONS

Means are used to determine significance for results displayed in Table 25. An (*) indicates significance at the .05 level and an (**) indicates significance at the .01 level. Statements with means significantly below 3.0 indicate agreement, and statements with means significantly greater than 3.0 indicate disagreement. Statements not significantly different from the mean indicate neutrality.

There are a few statements in which there are statistically significant differences in the responses between these two groups. First, there is a dichotomy in the perception of whether African Americans are the victims of an economic system that dictates both their ability to receive health services and the quality of their health (Q22). The African Americans tend to agree (mean = 2.385), but the Caucasians disagree (mean = 3.307).

They hold different views about whether the media care more about diseases that affect white people than about diseases that affect blacks (Q25). The African Americans believe the media are biased (mean = 2.725), but the Caucasians disagree (mean = 3.563).

TABLE 25
STATISTICAL COMPARISON OF AFRICAN AMERICAN AND CAUCASIAN MEANS

Statement	African Americans	Caucasians
Q15 We do not have a health care crisis in this country.	3.996**	3.807**
Q16 There is not much I can do to keep from getting sick.	3.371**	3.885**
Q17 I can't get health care because I have no transportation to and from a doctor's office, clinic, or hospital.	3.770**	3.974**
Q18 Support groups are important because many people can relate to others who are like themselves.	1.942**	1.918**
Q19 I am reluctant to obtain early treatment for illnesses because care is provided mainly by white medical personnel.	3.747**	4.026**
Q20 I only need to worry about today because the future will take care of itself.	3.767**	4.089**
Q21 Many doctors are prejudiced against African Americans.	3.241**	3.439**
Q22 African Americans are the victims of an economic system that dictates both their ability to receive health services and the quality of their health.	2.385**	3.307**
Q23 It is more important for an American health care system to give free medical care to the poor and disadvantaged than to give free care to middle and upper income citizens.	2.523**	2.725**
Q24 Getting the health care I need is usually too much trouble.	3.576**	3.714**
Q25 As long as a disease is hitting white people, the media care. But if it's hitting mainly African Americans, they are not going to worry about it too much.	2.725**	3.563**
Q26 The real key to good health is to lead a clean, moral life.	2.551**	2.851*

TABLE 25 *(continued)*

Statement	African Americans	Caucasians
Q27 If I can save money down the line, I might take preventive measures now to avoid the expense of having a heart attack and paying doctors bills or whatever.	1.961**	1.833**
Q28 It is appropriate to use newspapers to try to get information out about health risks such heart disease and diabetes.	2.453**	2.137**
Q29 If you have an important message about health care, put it on television.	2.121**	2.138**
Q30 If I need immediate medical care, I probably would go to a hospital emergency room rather than to a private physician.	2.580**	2.970
Q31 Illness can be a punishment from God.	3.798**	4.108**
Q32 The health care system makes me feel like I'm poor.	3.102	3.111
Q33 Physicians and health care practitioners need to respect the pride, values, and folkways of people they are trying to reach.	1.840**	1.852**
Q34 Community leaders (such as teachers and preachers) are important to the success of any health care campaign.	2.297**	2.226**
Q35 I believe that all Americans have a right—not a privilege—to health care.	1.712**	2.130*
Q36 If I'm not feeling well, I have no trouble finding time to go to the doctor.	2.724**	2.778**
Q37 Federal policies prohibiting discrimination in health service delivery should be enforced.	1.918**	2.045**
Q38 Lack of access to basic health care is an urgent social issue.	2.117**	2.315**
Q39 Any successful health campaign that could change behaviors would have to originate in my community, not at the state or national level.	2.799*	2.985
Q40 Health campaigns for particular diseases should emphasize that these are health care concerns for all people, rather than labeling them as just concerns for African Americans.	2.016**	2.007**

TABLE 25 *(continued)*

Statement		African Americans	Caucasians
Q41	Churches really have no role in promoting better physical health.	3.398**	3.370**
Q42	A health care system that gives everyone the help they need is never going to happen.	3.090	2.870
Q43	Access to health care and to the means of maintaining health are simply out of the reach of those not able to pay.	2.332**	2.681**
Q44	To reach minorities effectively with prevention information requires messages and programs that are tailored for and targeted to reach a specific audience.	2.310**	2.290**
Q45	I know all I need to know about how to stay well.	3.525**	3.496**
Q46	The ability of a doctor to help me depends in large part on my belief that the doctor will help me.	2.253**	2.319**
Q47	Illnesses are not discussed in my family.	3.856**	4.037**
Q48	People are more likely to participate when they are recognized as a person, rather than being labeled, isolated and separated into minority groups.	1.898**	1.896**
Q49	If you go to a hospital and they figure you may not have insurance or you're undercovered, they always make you wait. But, if you have insurance, they take you right in.	2.431**	3.052
Q50	Everyone does not have equal access to health care.	2.000**	2.193**
Q51	I take the time to read health stories in newspapers and magazines.	2.163**	2.130**
Q52	Preventive health efforts must be improved in disadvantaged areas.	1.813**	1.874**
Q53	The federal government's health policies are geared for the general population. They don't help minorities very much.	2.867	3.359**
Q54	Racial barriers to health care are not an issue.	3.333**	3.119

TABLE 25 *(continued)*

Statement		African Americans	Caucasians
Q55	I will go to a doctor only if I think something is wrong with my health.	3.051	2.678**
Q56	Rich people get better medical care than poor people.	2.020**	2.041**
Q57	My inclination is to stay away from doctors because you're not really sick until the doctor says you are.	3.883**	3.889**
Q58	The whole health care delivery system needs to be overhauled.	2.137**	2.422**
Q59	I have a great deal of pride in the American health care system.	2.805*	3.030
Q60	Minorities have not been taught how to use the health care system.	2.617**	3.052
Q61	The ultimate solution to providing adequate health care for African Americans is to educate enough black health care providers to do it.	2.543**	3.063
Q62	It doesn't matter to me whether doctors are black or white as long as they pay attention to my needs.	1.813**	1.770**
Q63	Blacks are more likely to die from diseases that can be cured or managed than are other minority groups and whites.	2.477**	2.810**

The Caucasians are neutral toward whether successful health campaign should originate at the community level, but the African Americans agree with this statement (mean = 2.799).

The African Americans agree that lack of insurance will mean long waits for medical care (mean = 2.431), while the Caucasians are neutral toward this statement (Q49).

Although the African Americans disagree that racial barriers to health care are not an issue (mean = 3.333), the Caucasians are neutral (Q54).

The Caucasians agree that they will go to the doctor only if they think something is wrong with their health (mean = 2.678), but the African Americans are neutral toward this statement (Q55).

The African Americans agree they have a great deal of pride in the American health care system (mean = 2.805), but the Caucasians are neutral (Q59).

The African Americans agree that minorities have not been taught how to use the health care system (mean = 2.617), but the Caucasians are neutral (Q59).

Although the Caucasians are neutral toward the statement that the ultimate solution to providing adequate health care for African Americans is to educate enough black health care providers to do it (Q61), African Americans agree with the statement (mean = 2.543).

MEDIA RELIANCE AND DEMOGRAPHIC COMPARISONS

To examine racial differences in regard to the remaining questions included in the telephone survey, crosstabulation tables using the Chi-Square test of statistical differences are used. Results that are significant to the .05 level are indicated below.

MEDIA RELIANCE DIFFERENCES

As other studies have suggested, the African Americans in this study watch more hours of television per week than the Caucasians in the sample do. A quarter of the African Americans view 26 hours or more of television a week, compared to 15% of the Caucasians (p=.00338).

Radio listenership is similar for the two groups. However, of 482 persons who listen to the radio, 69% of the African Americans, compared to 11% of the Caucasians listen to stations that program primarily for blacks (p=.00000).

TABLE 26
TELEVISION/RADIO HOURS PER WEEK

Group	Television Hours /Week	Radio Hours/Week
African American	21.5 N=252	15.4 N=257
Caucasians	16.7 N=270	14.9 N=268

Almost 74% of the Caucasians said they regularly subscribe to or read a newspaper, compared to 65% of the African Americans (p=.02345). Of the 365 persons who do read a newspaper, 57% of the African Americans, compared to 9% of the Caucasians, read a black newspaper (p=.00000).

SOURCES OF HEALTH INFORMATION

Because rank-ordering is very difficult to do in a telephone interview, respondents were read two lists, one of interpersonal health information sources and one of media health information sources. They were asked to give their No. 1 source from each list. There were no statistical differences between the groups in terms of interpersonal sources. Physicians are the No. 1 source for both groups.

TABLE 27
INTERPERSONAL SOURCES

Sources	Percentage	
	African American	Caucasian
Doctors	59.4%	53.5%
Nurses	5.1%	4.5%
Family members	14.2%	15.6%
Friends	5.9%	10.0%
Multiple sources	8.3%	7.8%
No sources	7.1%	8.6%
N=523		

However, there is a statistically significant difference between the two groups for media sources (p=.00456).

TABLE 28
MEDIA SOURCES

Sources	Percentage	
	African American	Caucasian
Newspapers	13.8%	23.5%
Magazines	16.7%	25.0%
Radio	6.1%	5.2%
Television	36.2%	28.4%
Medical publications	22.8%	15.7%
Multiple sources	1.2%	.4%
No sources	3.3%	1.9%
N=514		

HEALTH ARTICLE READERSHIP

Caucasians are much more likely than African Americans to say they read health articles in newspapers and magazines (p=.00284). Of the Caucasians, 52% read these types of articles regularly, 39% read them occasionally, and 9% rarely or never read them. Of the African Americans, 43% regularly read

health articles, 39% occasionally read them, and 18% never read them
(p=.00284).

There were readership differences between the races for only four
specific types of health articles: diabetes, sickle cell anemia, child and infant
health, and AIDS.

TABLE 29
HEALTH ARTICLE READERSHIP BY GROUP

Article Type	Percentage	
	African American	Caucasian
Diet & Nutrition	82.4%	84.1%
N=526 (p=.61185)		
Exercise	79.6%	81.5%
N=525 (p=.58761)		
Diabetes	75.4%	67.0%
N=526 (p=.03464)		
Heart/ High Blood Pressure	86.7%	84.1%
N=526 (p=.39110)		
Glaucoma/Eye Disease	61.9%	58.1%
N=527 (p=.38371)		
Sickle Cell Anemia	68.6%	32.6%
N=525 (p=.00000)		
Cancer	85.5%	85.9%
N=526 (p=.90110)		
Elderly Diseases	70.7%	67.4%
N=526 (p=.41395)		
Child/Infant Health	67.5%	51.1%
N=525 (p=.00014)		
Stress	83.6%	84.1%
N=526 (p=.88109)		
AIDS	85.2%	71.9%
N=526 (p=.00021)		
General Health	87.1%	90.0%
N=525 (p=.28976)		

There is no differences between the races concerning the general
believability of newspaper and magazine health articles.

TABLE 30
HEALTH ARTICLE BELIEVABILITY

Level	Percentage	
	African American	Caucasian
Generally believes	37.8%	42.8%
Usually questions	36.7%	37.5%
Depends on source	25.5%	19.7%
N=520		

HEALTH STATUS

There are no differences in the percentage of those who currently smoke (about 25% of each group), who have quit within the past two years (between 6% and 9%), and who never smoked or have not smoked in recent years (about two-thirds of both groups).

However, there was a difference in drinking habits between the two groups (p=.01311). Thirty percent of the Caucasians, compared to 20% of the African Americans, said they currently drink at least once a week; about 10% of both groups said they have quit drinking or reduced the amount they drink; and 70% of African Americans, compared to 59% of the Caucasians said they rarely or never drink.

Eighty-six percent of both groups said within the past two years, they have taken action to improve their own or their family's health. The form this action has taken varies, however. Almost 86% of the Caucasians, compared to 76% of the African Americans, said they had modified their diets (p=.00736). About 60% of both groups said they increased the amount they exercise, and about 65% of both groups have reduced stress.

TABLE 31
LIFESTYLE CHANGES BY GROUP

Change	Percentage	
	African American	Caucasian
Modified diet N=492 (p=.00736)	76.3%	85.7%
Increased exercise N=519 (p=.59308)	59.1%	61.4%
Reduced stress N=514 (p=.57055)	66.4%	64.0%

HEALTH STATUS COMPARISONS

The African Americans in the sample are more likely to have high blood pressure (32% compared to 21%, p=.00491). Otherwise, there were no significant differences in health status.

TABLE 32
CHRONIC DISEASE BY GROUP

Disease	Percentage	
	African American	Caucasian
Diabetes	8.7%	9.1%
N=514 (p=.57055)		
Glaucoma/Eye Disease	5.9%	6.4%
N=518 (p=.80080)		
High Blood Pressure	31.5%	20.7%
N=520 (p=.00491)		
Heart/Coronary Artery Disease	7.9%	9.7%
N=521 (p=.45356)		
High Cholesterol	14.2%	19.9%
N=508 (p=.08537)		
Lung/Respiratory Disease	8.7%	9.0%
N=521 (p=.91688)		
Cancer	3.6%	5.6%
N=521 (p=.27532)		
Stroke/Brain Impairment	2.0%	1.5%
N=524 (p=.67651)		
Arthritis	23.5%	25.7%
N=516 (p=.57014)		

The Caucasians in the sample are significantly more likely to have a family physician (90% compared to 83%, p=.01570).

MEDICARE/MEDICAID AND INSURANCE STATUS

Although 73% of the Caucasians and 65% of the African Americans said they use neither Medicare nor Medicaid, there are differences among those using these government programs (p=.00004). Twenty percent of the Caucasians, compared to 15% of the African Americans, use Medicare, although 13% of the African Americans, compared to 3% of the Caucasians use Medicaid. About 7% of the African Americans, compared to 5% of the Caucasians, use both programs.

The Caucasians in the sample are much more likely to have private or group medical insurance that covers hospitalization and/or visits to doctors (p=.00000). Eighty-seven percent have insurance, compared to 68% of the African Americans.

KNOWLEDGE AND ATTITUDES TOWARD THE CLINTON HEALTH PLAN

Subjects were asked about their general knowledge of the health care reform package that President Bill Clinton presented to Congress for consideration. There is a significant difference in response between the two groups. Of the African Americans, 20% said they know nothing about the proposal, 28% said they have limited knowledge, 46% said they know something about the proposal but may not understand everything about it, and 7% said they are knowledgeable about the proposal. In contrast, only 8% of the Caucasians said they know nothing about the proposal, 32% said they have limited knowledge, 48% said they know something about the proposal but may not understand everything about it, and 12% said they are knowledgeable about the proposal (p=.00031).

TABLE 33
KNOWLEDGE OF CLINTON PLAN BY GROUP

Knowledge	Percentage	
	African American	Caucasian
Knowledgeable	6.7%	12.3%
Knows something	45.9%	47.6%
Limited knowledge	27.8%	32.3%
Knows nothing	19.6%	7.8%
N=524		

There also is a statistically significant difference between the races in regard to support for Clinton's plan to guarantee health insurance to everyone (.00000). Even though a higher percentage of African Americans said they know nothing about Clinton's plan, more than three-fourths (78%) of them said they favor guaranteed health insurance.

TABLE 34
SUPPORT FOR CLINTON'S PLAN BY GROUP

Support	Percentage	
	African American	Caucasian
Favors	77.6%	51.1%
Opposes	8.3%	34.4%
Undecided	14.4%	14.4%
N=524		

DEMOGRAPHICS

As expected, the education level between the two groups varies considerably (p=.00000). Fifteen percent of the African Americans, compared to 4% of the Caucasians, have not graduated from high school. (In fact, 5% of the African Americans, compared to less than 1% of the Caucasians had less than a ninth grade education.) A quarter of the Caucasians, compared to 14% of the African Americans, are college graduates; and 18% of the Caucasians, compared to 4% of the African Americans, have advanced degrees (master's, Ph.D., or professional).

The African Americans in this sample tend to be younger than the Caucasians (p=.00812). Almost 18% of the African Americans, compared to 8% of the Caucasians are between the ages of 18 to 24. Conversely, 34% of the Caucasians, compared to 26% of the African Americans, are 55 or older.

There is no significant difference in the percentage of both groups that are currently working in a health-related field. Because only 62 persons (30 Caucasians and 32 African Americans) work in health-related field, the sample is too small to determine statistical significance. However, the Caucasians in the sample are much more likely to be registered nurses or administrators than the African Americans, while the majority of black health care workers are nurses aids, technicians, and members of hospital cleaning staffs.

African Americans are almost twice as likely as the Caucasians in this sample to be unmarried (.00000). Of the African Americans, 41% are single, 11% are widowed, and 20% are divorced or separated, while only 27% are married. Of the Caucasians, 26% are single, 7% are widowed, and 10% are divorced or separated, while 57% are married.

African Americans reported a higher number of household members compared to Caucasian households (p=.00052). One-third have four or more persons in the household, compared to 20% of the Caucasians.

Income levels also are significantly different (p=.00000). Twenty-seven percent of the African Americans, compared to 8% of the Caucasians have total annual household incomes of $10,000 or below. A quarter of the black households, compared to 14% of the white households, have incomes between $11,000 and $19,999 a year. Conversely, 37% of the white households, compared to 11% of the black households have total yearly incomes of $46,000 or more.

The University of Missouri-St. Louis Public Policy Research Center used the 1990 U.S. Census to assure that the St. Louis sample represents the population and then projected these results to the samples in Kansas City and Baton Rouge. When the adult African American and Caucasians populations are considered (18+), 43% are black and 57% are white. In this sample, 49% are black and 51% are white. As previously mentioned, African Americans were deliberately over-sampled to provide more reliable comparisons between the races.

There is no statistically significant difference in the male/female split of either sample. One-third of the African American sample is male, compared to 38% of the Caucasian sample. Of the total African American population, 42% are male and 58% are female. Of the total Caucasian population, 45% are male and 55% are female. Females are over-represented, but this is not unexpected in a telephone survey because a higher percentage of females answer the telephone and are more likely to participate.

CHAPTER X

Implications for Communication and Marketing Theories:
An African American Perspective

This study has shown that a multi-dimensional approach is desirable when planning health campaigns. Planners first should be familiar with communication theory because if there is no understanding of how individuals obtain and use health care information, there can be no valid method of promoting changes in behavior. Further, this study has demonstrated that Q methodology is an effective way to segment a mass audience attitudinally. Also, a step is taken to increase the potency of Q methodology by devising a technique to extend Q sort results to a large, random sample of the mass audience. This permits the evaluation of different attitude clusters found within the African American audience rather than relying on the traditional demographic approach that often assumes all African Americans are similar and can be reached with a single approach.

Once the audience is segmented and described, strategies for the effective planning and dispersing of health messages can be devised. Social marketing techniques combine communication theory and marketing theory to help create effective messages and emphasizes the importance of message placement (through the media and/or interpersonal channels). Social marketing also emphasizes the need for constant testing and evaluation of all campaign efforts.

Many of the issues discussed in this book were developed primarily from focus group research. The author was initially struck by responses from African Americans discussing health issues that seemed more cultural than economic in nature. For example, many of the participants from the diabetes support group in St. Louis mentioned that their parents had not discussed their illness and that, as a consequence, they did not know that they personally were at risk for developing diabetes. Also, for the most part, their diabetes had not been diagnosed in a routine screening. Most had become seriously ill or were being treated for another, often unrelated, illness before their diabetes was diagnosed. A few members of this group also were convinced that black physicians are more likely than white physicians to screen their patients for diabetes and other diseases prevalent in African Americans.

FINDINGS

This study developed five hypotheses to guide the investigation of attitudes about health care. The hypotheses and the results of their testing are summarized below:

H1:   Attitudes about health care are not unidimensional. The target audience can be segmented into definable groups of people who hold similar attitudes.

Members of each group will have attitudes that are distinct from every other group.

The target audience was segmented into five Q types—The Equalizers, The Adjusters, The Preventers, The Empathizers, and The Fixers—each of which has a distinct pattern of attitudes. Further, these types were successfully extended to the larger audience through the telephone survey and cluster analysis. Each segment emphasizes to some extent different health care issues and barriers. Thus, H1 is confirmed.

H2:   Not all African Americans think alike about health care. African American attitudes about health care will be represented by more than one clearly identifiable target audience segment.

Although there is evidence that racial experience does assist in forming attitudes, African Americans are found in every Q type and in every cluster. Therefore, there is no universal "black" attitude. H2 is confirmed.

H3:   Media exposure and reliance patterns will not be uniform across all segments. Some audience segments are expected to be exposed more to print media (newspapers and magazines) than to broadcast media (radio and television), while the reverse will be true for other segments.

There are (predominately black) Q types and clusters that are primarily dependent on broadcast media, while other (predominately white) types are as dependent or more dependent on print media. Also, black media are used by large segments of the African American audience, while Caucasians are much less likely to pay attention to media targeted toward blacks. H3 is confirmed.

H4: Media sources will be more influential than interpersonal sources in the delivery of health care messages.

Physicians are the No. 1 source of health information for every Q cluster. However, a higher percentage of participants in the telephone survey indicate they do not have an interpersonal source (ranging from 6% to 9% across clusters) compared to the media sources (ranging from 1% to 6% across clusters). The Q sorts indicate that The Adjusters and The Fixers are more dependent on the media and less dependent on doctors for information than the other Q types. However, African Americans, in general, indicate they discuss illnesses in their families. As stated, H4 is not supported because although media sources are pervasive, interpersonal sources (especially physicians and family members) obviously exert a strong influence on the communication of health information.

H5: Concerns about the health care system and recognition of barriers to obtaining health care will not be uniform across all segments.

The Preventers prove in both the Q sorts and telephone survey that they are oblivious to many of barriers that hinder adequate health care. However, even when barriers are recognized, The Fixers focus mainly on barriers related to poverty, while The Equalizers and The Adjusters emphasize both economic and access barriers. The Equalizers and The Adjusters want to make access equal for all, but The Fixers think more radical health reform is needed. H5 is confirmed.

COMMUNICATION THEORY

Communication theory supports expectations that cultural, economic, and educational differences will influence communication. Starting with the concept of a "mass audience," communication theory offers several reasons why there may be communication problems in transmitting health care information. Discussed at length in Chapter III, barriers to communication include various ways individuals ignore or filter messages. These theories also examine mass media effects and ways in which the media are more likely to bring about changes in opinions, attitudes, and to a lesser extend behaviors.

The discussion focuses on two- and multi-step flow processes, dissonance, selectivity of various types, and social categories, modeling, meaning, and consistency theories that consider broadly how messages move through channels and how receivers (individuals) may receive, avoid, or block the message. Uses and gratification, knowledge gap, diffusion, and network analysis theories are more concerned with how the audience, either active or passive, reacts to messages. Individuals within a mass audience may, for example, use the media toward pleasurable ends (as play), may adopt and pass on messages or innovations through networks, or may avoid media messages and become less knowledgeable than others in society. Agenda setting examines how the media help set the public agenda, increase knowledge, and influence opinion leaders. All of these provide some explanations why African Americans may not receive, absorb, or pass along health care information in the same way that Caucasians or other minority groups do.

Each of these communication theories has some limitations. For example, diffusion theory focuses on the characteristics of an adopter and stresses the source of the information (media, opinion leader, etc.) but does not delve into the characteristics of the source that makes communication most effective. That is, the media are given much importance in the role of disseminating information and creating awareness, but there is no study of how the media accomplish this role. Also, it primarily is concerned with the dissemination of an innovation, a new idea or method, whereas much health care information is not innovative. For example, people have known for a long time that smoking has been linked to lung cancer and other ailments, but many have not adopted the idea that cigarettes can kill them. Competing ideas (cigarette advertising versus stop smoking campaigns) that advocate different behaviors can hinder the diffusion process.

Agenda setting and two-step or multi-step flow theories begin to examine how the media influence a mass audience. They dismiss the idea of a "magic bullet" effect and look instead toward communication networks. The media affect opinion leaders who in turn persuade people in their sphere of influence. However, these theories do not emphasize the individual's internal decision-making process, values, and lifestyle.

The knowledge gap hypothesis explains why the poor and disadvantaged are likely to take less notice of information available than those with higher incomes and more education. But, it does not explain how people can form a viewpoint about issues without much knowledge of them. For example, even though there definitely is a knowledge gap concerning the Clinton health plan, people still tended to support or oppose it on the basis of what they personally want or what they assume the plan contains. In other words, opinions have been formed without a knowledge base. This hypothesis does little to explain how that process occurs. Also, there can be other gaps, such as lack of information or available health care services, that persist even if people are motivated and knowledgeable.

Uses and gratifications theory brings in the dimension of consumer needs and the satisfaction consumers receive from communication. The difficulty, of course, is determining on a mass scale which messages will meet needs and whether people will find positive health care actions (such as exercising and giving up cigarettes) as gratifying as unhealthy habits (drinking, smoking, etc.). Also, there is the problem of determining whether the audience really is active or if at some points in the communication process some or all parts of the audience are passive. It seems likely in the case of health care communication that people with a particular illness will actively seek information about the illness while those who are healthy may not have any particular reason to attend to health care messages.

Network analysis moves ahead to pull many of these elements together and to look at communication as a system. It explains how communication works in specific communities where people can act as both transmitters and receivers of information. However, it is more difficult to examine how this model might work when a mass audience is involved or what role the mass media might have in it (other than as an information source). The difficulty with convergence is how to identify cliques and measure communication links. This is especially difficult if the researcher is trying to analyze a community with several thousand members, such as an inner-city community, as opposed to a village of a few hundred. This research has attempted to describe a model that will divide either the large inner-city area or the small village into attitudinal cliques (Q types). Once these cliques have been defined, then it is possible to do a large sample survey to determine the relative representation of each clique (Q type) within the total population. Although Rogers and Kincaid are looking at interpersonal communication in relatively small communities, it is likely that larger versions of their networks exist. For example, African American newspaper publishers have their own network of friends and acquaintances with whom they communicate and from whom they receive feedback. But, a black newspaper circulating within the community forms a large-scale system whereby information is transmitted along a "link." Feedback is received in the form of letters-to-the-editor, telephone calls, and casual contact between the newspaper's publisher and reporters and community members. The system may expand to include local ministers who may influence the religion page found in many black newspapers and politicians who influence the political coverage in the newspaper. News coverage and editorial comment can provide feedback to the minister and the politician who in turn communicate with their congregations and constituents. Members of congregations communicate to family members. Before long, information has been passed along both formally and informally to many members of the community.

MARKETING THEORY

Marketing theorists are even more concerned with behavior change than are communication theorists because the end goal of marketing activities is to produce a behavior (purchasing a product, viewing a corporation or brand in a favorable light, adopting an idea or desired mode of action, etc.). Communication theorists by and large are pessimistic that behavior change can be brought about through mass media communication, but marketing theorists are determined that behavior change is possible, although they are reluctant to rely solely on the mass media to effect such change.

First, marketers see the need for "campaigns," not single communications. This term implies that there must be a number of "assaults" from a number of angles. Merely placing one advertisement on television, for example, cannot be expected to effect a behavior change. Marketers are concerned with audience segmentation because they know that one consumer is not necessarily like another. Therefore, ways must be found to first identify and then understand the various segments, or publics, that must then have communications tailored to their needs and perspectives. Social marketing is based on the assumption that ideas that foster the public good, in this case health care, can be "sold" in the same way that products are sold.

At its most basic, social marketing is concerned with implementation of campaign activities and evaluation of the effectiveness of those activities. At its most complex, social marketing uses communication and social-psychological theories to develop programs, and marketing techniques to develop messages and implement the program. In addition to the mass media, social marketers also use local organizations and interpersonal networks to influence behavior change. Social marketing has among its goals bridging gaps in comprehension, awareness, knowledge, and behavior. Consensus building is another of the goals of social marketing. Beyond reliance on media, social marketers will look for opinion leaders, influential people, and members of organizations within a target community who will "buy into" the social marketing agenda and help further the cause or causes being promoted.

An obvious component of social marketing is advertising theory. Social marketers are well aware of the problem of clutter that makes it difficult for consumers to "weed out" messages meant for them. Social marketers also view the media as impersonal. Just as an advertising executive will choose the media that provides the best "reach" for an ad, the social marketer will select the media that are best suited to the campaign.

Finally, the social marketer knows the value of evaluation. Every aspect of the campaign will be tested and evaluated if possible. Messages, publication content and design, and advertising messages and presentation will all be pre-tested. Recall tests and other methods of assessing impact will be undertaken. Here, the methods of communications theorists, advertising theorists, and marketing theorists will overlap. Such methods as focus groups, telephone surveys, and personal interviews will be used to plan and evaluate communication efforts.

RESEARCH TECHNIQUES

One of the major techniques for studying communication is network analysis. However, such analysis can be time-consuming, or even impossible in large communities. Some shortcuts are possible by combining Q methodology with other ways of gathering information. For example, survey instruments for this study included questions about both interpersonal and media sources of information. It would be possible to devise Q sorts that would be administered to presumed community leaders (physicians, ministers, politicians, educators, etc.). Additional sorts with various members of the target community then could be obtained and compared with the leaders' sorts. This method would determine which leaders best match the community (or segments of the community). These leaders then should be persuaded to assist with the planning and implementing of the social marketing campaign.

Focus groups and large sample surveys can be used to refine the findings and test whether chosen opinion leaders are acceptable to either segments or the total community. Brenner also has demonstrated how Q methodology can be used to explain the failure to adopt an innovation and how it is in sync with the convergence model (measuring connectedness, integration, diversity, and openness).

Combining Q methodology with large sample surveying techniques can provide a great deal of information about the individuals who make up the larger community as this study demonstrates. A review of medical literature confirmed that African Americans are generally in poorer health than any other group in America. The documentation of the many health problems that are more acute in the black population have been summarized previously, with most researchers concluding that if cures are found for poverty, the health of African Americans would automatically improve. While accepting the validity of this assertion, the author continues to have concerns about whether physicians and researchers have been too quick to blame poverty while often dismissing or not even considering cultural barriers that may not be dependent upon economic status. Because cultural differences can interfere with communication, it seems reasonable to examine attitudes and behaviors together rather than merely examining behaviors or outcomes as much of the medical literature tends to do.

Rather than comparing black and white rates of hospitalization, emergency room visits, or mortality and morbidity rates, this researcher undertook a study that examines both attitudes and behaviors in tandem. That is, rather than merely looking at statistics concerning emergency room visits, this researcher first asked whether subjects would be more likely to go to an emergency room than to see a private doctor, whether they believe they have access to the health care system, and whether the American system is meeting their needs, etc., and then determined whether they have personal physicians, whether they have been hospitalized, whether they have insurance, and whether they have made lifestyles changes to improve their health, and so on. The main object is to determine whether there are, in fact, distinct differences between African Americans and Caucasians in attitudes and behaviors that account for some of the discrepancies in health status. Hypothesizing that this would, indeed, be the case, the author then looked to communication theory and marketing theory to first explain these differences and to then devise ways to overcome them if they were found to exist.

Social marketing and advertising theory focus on the receivers of information. They advocate the use of market segmentation and individual behaviors. They have relied primarily on psychographics—VALS or AIO—and demographics to accomplish segmentation. However, these theories often spend more time in discussing how to formulate an effective message than they do in determining which media channels and interpersonal channels are the most effective dissemination methods.

COMMUNICATION AXIOMS

This research suggests several axioms that should be considered when communicating with an African American population. The first, and most important axiom, is that rather than thinking of African Americans as a single mass audience, the communicator must understand there are multiple segments (publics, clusters, Q types, cliques, etc.) within the larger population. These segments should be defined along attitudinal lines rather than along demographic lines. This does not mean that economic status and education levels should be ignored because both can affect attitude formation. But, relying solely on demographics will falsely group people into clusters that may have little in common attitudinally. As communication research implies and marketing research expects, changing attitudes can change behavior. Therefore, it is far more important to identify and group people with similar attitudes than it is to group people with similar demographics.

Although social marketing recognizes the importance of examining the audience on various levels, Grunig falls short of being able to suggest a methodology for examining his "innermost nest" of individual communication behaviors and effects or his second nest of "publics" that consists of individuals who communicate and behave in similar ways. This research clearly shows that Q methodology can do both.

The second axiom is that mass media alone will likely not bring about the desired behavior change. African Americans are more reliant on television than on the print media. Television as a channel of information has become more and more fragmented with the growth in cable and eventually smaller and cheaper satellite dishes that will literally put hundreds of channels at the viewer's fingertips. Consequently, even if the majority of African Americans are tuned in to television, the odds of them tuning into the same channel at the same time become lower every year. Caucasians are more likely than African Americans to read health articles in newspapers and magazines, although African Americans show more interest in articles about diseases that disproportionately affect them: diabetes, sickle cell anemia, and AIDS. But, there is still a distrust of media medical articles, with many African Americans and Caucasians saying they either usually question the health articles they read or they judge their accuracy based on the source of the information. Certainly, this research demonstrates that using black newspapers, magazines, and radio to disperse health care messages certainly will increase the odds that African Americans will be exposed to these messages.

The third axiom is that campaign efforts at the community level will be more successful if local opinion leaders are involved. Much of the power in a black community rests with ministers, politicians, physicians, and educators, often male. As a white, female researcher, it was important for the author to use the existing power structure to gain the cooperation of African

American subjects. Even so, there was suspicion about the research motives and limits to the cooperation extended. (The Black Health Care Coalition, for example, assisted with one focus group but declined to submit questions for the Kansas City portion of the telephone survey.) Outsiders can be involved, but they cannot affect change or mount a successful campaign without at least the appearance of local sponsorship and cooperation. The leadership aspects of black media owners should not be overlooked either. Focus groups, for example, indicated that media owners and ministers are among the major opinion leaders within most black communities. Health care campaign planners should most certainly include both local publishers or media owners and ministers in message planning and delivery.

The third axiom is that messages targeted toward African Americans must be carefully planned and tested to avoid inadvertently presenting the wrong message. Some groups within the black community resent being viewed as victims. For example, although there is high interest in information about AIDS, many African Americans will resist messages that depict them as victims of AIDS, particularly if acquiring AIDS is in any way linked to black stereotypes (multiple sex partners, drug abuse, etc.). Conversely, some do view themselves as victims, either because the economic system makes health care unobtainable or because they have not been taught to use the health care system to their advantage. In short, some avoid seeking health care because they have encountered, or at least they fear they will encounter, racism within the health care system. Even terms such as "African American" and "black" are not accepted universally within the black community and carry negative or even racist connotations for some segments. For this research, for example, one woman in a focus group said that she had never lived in Africa and, therefore, was most definitely *not* an African American. In conversations, however, many refer to members of their race as "blacks." One person responding to a mail survey even listed his race as "Negro." The point is that even "African American," a term considered politically correct in many circles, is a negative term to some. One method of overcoming these difficulties is to use a multi-cultural approach with the aim of bringing people together rather than labeling and separating them into groups.

The fourth axiom is that there is a fatalism within the black community that must be recognized before it can be overcome. One of the main reasons African Americans may avoid the health care system or chose emergency rooms over private physicians is that some see little point in preventive action when they live totally in the present without much thought of the future. If they are healthy today, they are not going to worry about being sick tomorrow. For example, many of the African Americans in this study expressed a sense of pessimism that they can control the state of their own health. If they are fatalistic about their health (i.e., if I am destined to get sick, I will), they are less likely to exercise, eat properly, and get preventive health care (flu shots, blood pressure checks, and the like). Messages about health care aimed at this particular segment must find stimuli other than "an ounce of prevention is worth a pound of cure." Possibly an economic approach, such as "seeing a doctor today may save you thousands of dollars tomorrow" will be effective. But, even better is a message that urges people to check their blood pressure because "today you might be sick and not even know it."

The fifth axiom is that having black health care professionals available is important to many in the black community. Even though they agree that the color of their doctors is less important than the attitude of their doctors, many still would prefer to have a doctor who "speaks their language." They may not think it is necessary to have a black doctor because many have never been given that choice. The bottom line is that communication between physician and patient needs to be improved, and it needs to be improved along cultural lines. Affluent, highly educated white physicians simply have trouble "converging" with poor or not highly educated black patients, and vice versa. For example, some focus group participants said they did not want a doctor to give them orders about their health. They need to feel that they are making choices for themselves. This can frustrate doctors who believe they know what is best for the patient, so "why don't my patients just do what I tell them to." Black doctors may be more sensitive to subtle communication differences. It may be necessary for a campaign to include messages that give patients tips about communicating with doctors. (Medical school and in-service training for physicians need similar components.)

The sixth axiom is related to the fifth. The health care planner must recognize that African Americans are more likely to get information from their physicians than they are from family and friends or media sources. Thus, physicians of all races, especially African American physicians, should be included in any health care effort aimed at African Americans. They may require specialized training or at least need some materials designed for them that they can pass along to patients. Also, physicians who work in a clinic or emergency room setting should be aware that many African American patients do not see the same doctor on subsequent visits. They are less likely than Caucasians to have family doctors. So, every physician must see dispensing basic health care information as much a part of his or her job as dispensing medicine.

The seventh axiom is that African Americans have experienced and, therefore, recognize more barriers to health care than do Caucasians. Many of the Caucasians included in this study simply are oblivious to barriers because they have never lacked for transportation, for insurance, or for the means to pay health care costs. They give little thought to other segments of the population who may face these barriers. However, those who have encountered them understand that there is unequal access to health care. A necessary part of any effective health care campaign must be identifying barriers to health care and to find ways to overcome or at least mitigate these barriers before behavior will change.

The eighth axiom is that racial experience has an impact on attitudes toward health and the health care system. This is most in evidence by the fact that two of the Q types, one predominately black and the other predominately white, hold many similar attitudes but often diverge when statements refer directly to experiences and matters of race. Campaign planners must be sensitive to racial experiences and learn how to use them to encourage behavior change rather than to create unintentional attitudinal barriers to health care.

The ninth axiom is that even though there is statistical evidence that African Americans and Caucasians receive unequal treatment once they are in the health care system, neither blacks nor whites seem aware of possible racist attitudes and practices among health care providers. Possibly this is related to the fatalistic views of black patients (they expect poor outcomes, so they are less aggressive in demanding tests and treatments). Another possibility is that this type of racism exists at the unconscious level. Physicians do not consciously decide to withhold treatment, but they may assume that the patient can't afford it or won't want it and, therefore, does not recommend effective but very expensive courses of treatment.

VALUE OF THIS RESEARCH

How then has this research contributed to both communication and marketing theory? Beyond the testing of the hypotheses that underlie this research, a method has been found to effectively group the mass audience into the attitude "segments" (Q types) that are so important to social marketing efforts, to describe those segments, and then to determine the likely proportion of each segment within a mass audience (clusters). This research ties together Q methodology, communication theory (most notably diffusion and network analysis), and social marketing. This research has been uniquely concerned with examining attitudes of African Americans (compared with Caucasians) along with current behaviors to determine how best to affect future behavior change.

While diffusion theory explains how people adopt innovations or ideas that lead to behavior change, network analysis views communication as a function of a system with identifiable cliques, specialized communication roles, communication structural indexes, and communication links. Diffusion theory predicts that those who lack economic means and education are not likely to be opinion leaders. It also relies heavily on the mass media as the purveyor of information necessary to stimulate the adoption curve. This researcher must argue that although the tenets of diffusion should be kept in mind while planning a health care campaign (particularly the five characteristics of an innovation: relative advantage, compatibility, complexity, trialability, and observability), this model will not be as effective as the convergence model in planning health care campaigns because it is difficult to reach African Americans and stimulate the adoption curve through the mass media alone.

Convergence is the ultimate goal of health campaigns. Convergence requires a communication network made up of individuals, groups, and media. The difficulty with convergence is how to identify cliques and measure communication links. This is especially difficult if the researcher is trying to analyze a community with several thousand members, such as an inner-city community, as opposed to a village of a few hundred. This research has attempted to describe a model that will divide either the large inner-city area or the small village into attitudinal cliques (Q types). Once these cliques have been defined, then it is possible to do a large sample survey to determine the relative representation of each clique (Q type) within the total population.

IMPLICATIONS FOR COMMUNICATION THEORY AND SOCIAL MARKETING

What then are the implications of this study for communication theory and social marketing? The elements of communication and social marketing theory can come together in a marketing plan. Broadly, the main categories of analysis are the communicator, the content of the communication, the audience, and the actual responses made by the audience. Social marketing defines several steps within these areas that need special attention, and communication theory suggests ways to devise messages and plan the distribution of them. Q methodology provides a means of audience segmentation and campaign evaluation.

STRATEGIES

Health campaigns have been criticized for not focusing on behavior and for assuming that changing behavior is an easy task. Often there is over-reliance on the mass media while interpersonal contact is overlooked or at least not used to its potential. There also is a gap between what people say and what people do, often making it difficult to accurately assess the underlying attitudes and barriers that prevent positive courses of action. Also, health campaigns often are designed from the provider's point of view rather than from the target audience's or consumer's point of view.

Marketing concepts integrated with social influence theories can overcome many of these weaknesses. It is important to understand the audience and to attempt to determine how to make a passive audience more attentive and how to let an active audience know when and how to obtain health care services. This has been accomplished in this research by first examining the attitudes of the individual, then grouping individuals into similar attitude factors and clusters, and finally describing those segments in terms of demographics, psychographics, and communication networks. Communication networks are examined in terms of which mass media are depended upon the most, the No. 1 source of interpersonal information, and the role of churches and community efforts in a health care campaign. Media and interpersonal influences have been studied together because they are interactive.

This research has attempted to bring communication theories and marketing theories together primarily within the framework of Q methodology and social marketing because they attempt to combine market segmentation, message design, media selection, and community networks in campaign development. This model also offers a strong emphasis on evaluation and research techniques.

This researcher argues that each of the above theories offers aspects of the communication process that are important to a health care campaign. By remembering marketing's reliance on product, price, promotion, and place, and looking to diffusion theory to predict how a message or idea might be received and adopted, the campaign can be better planned and executed. Emphasis must also be placed on both the psychological process and the cultural processes involved in communication. Examining the way in which people select the messages they attend to and keeping a consistency in messages that reduces cognitive dissonance. Modeling theory also can help determine message content and can provide a visual context for desired behavior.

The power of the media to disseminate messages, help people put in context the importance of issues, and to influence opinions and attitudes should be used. In this case, the researcher suggests that the black media have not been used to its potential to reach African Americans and to set a health care agenda for them. However, this research also shows that the media alone are not sufficient to actually accomplish behavior change. It is important to include opinion leaders, social groups, and health care professionals if the campaign is to accomplish behavior change.

The final section suggests how to put together a marketing plan that targets African Americans.

THE COMMUNICATOR

In this case the communicator is any individual or group who designs and carries out a health campaign. Obviously, the communicator—in this case, the source of the message—is extremely important and must be credible. Nearly a quarter of those interviewed in the telephone survey indicated they evaluate the credibility of health care messages based on the source of the message. Consequently, any source of a health campaign should be perceived as credible. If the source has a credibility problem, then that image has to be improved before maximum campaign effectiveness can be achieved. Additionally, in as far as possible, the outlets for the campaign messages, i.e., newspapers, television, and radio, should be viewed as credible by the intended audience. A campaign to lower cholesterol originating from the American Heart Association, for example, will be perceived as more credible than one that originates from an association with no prior name identification.

IDENTIFYING HEALTH PROBLEMS

Medical research shows that African Americans face serious problems with high blood pressure, glaucoma, and diabetes, among other diseases. There are few if any initial symptoms for these diseases, which means that routine screenings are necessary. So, for the purposes of this discussion, increasing voluntary screenings will be the example used as the impetus for the health campaign.

ESTABLISHING PRIORITIES

The focus of health campaigns should be kept as narrow as possible to avoid confusing or conflicting messages or campaign elements. Because the focus is narrow and because funding will undoubtedly be limited, any effective campaign must set priorities. These priorities include identifying target audiences, identifying attitudes and opinions, planning messages, and planning message dispersion. In the example of planning a campaign to increase screening participation, it is necessary to prioritize which type of screening will be emphasized or which screening sites will be promoted first. If clinics are placed in African American churches, community centers, or public housing complexes, then an awareness campaign will be the first priority followed by a behavior change campaign. Ultimately, additional components, such as urging the adoption of low-fat diets, aerobic exercise, or reliance on a personal physician rather than an emergency room, can be added.

IDENTIFYING TARGET AUDIENCES

Much of this research has been concerned with identifying target audiences. The main argument is that it is not adequate to separate the mass audience along racial or demographic lines alone. To develop the most effective campaign, attitudes have to be determined. Focus groups and Q methodology are effective tools for accomplishing this. The previous chapters have illustrated how self-referent statements can be obtained, then used to form a Q sample that leads to identifying Q types. These statements can then be used in a large-sample survey to determine the likely percentage of the mass audience that each type represents.

Of course, it is useful to determine the demographic makeup of each type because some campaigns simply must be carried out along demographic lines. For example, a campaign aimed at teen-age mothers will be structured differently from a campaign aimed at older, working mothers. Above all, this research has demonstrated that race plays an important role in the formation of attitudes. But, even though there are distinct racial patterns, there also are several levels at which attitudes of both races overlap and other factors such as income and education become important in defining the target group. Although there are differences between African Americans and Caucasians, there also are definable segments within the African American population. Education levels, income levels, gender, and even geographic location can influence attitudes. Therefore, it is necessary to further differentiate the attitude clusters found within the African American population. Q methodology may be the only available vehicle for accomplishing this task.

IDENTIFYING MESSAGE ACTIONS

Above all, messages should be tailored to specific interests, needs, values, and beliefs of the various audience segments identified through focus groups and Q sorts. In this case, at least five different messages should be considered, one tailored toward each of the five Q types (or clusters). If funds are in short supply, then the best approach is to look for attitudes that cut across the types or can appeal to the types that account for the largest percentage of the total mass audience. For example, a multi-cultural message approach would likely appeal to both The Equalizers and The Adjusters because the main difference in these groups involves race-specific experiences. The best solution would be to develop one basic message but tailor its presentation differently for each type. For example, one television commercial should feature an African American spokesperson, and the second commercial should feature a white spokesperson. However, it also is possible to create one message with both black and white spokespersons together. At any rate, it is important to avoid the "one message fits all" approach.

Second, the literacy level of the target audience must be considered so that messages are not too complicated or too patronizing. We can assume that in part, illiteracy will be tied to lower education rates. Also, isolating those who said they do not read newspapers or magazines can be a good indication that a segment of the target audience cannot be reached through written communication. Consequently, messages designed for low literacy groups should rely heavily on pictures, and television and radio messages should be included.

The messages should, if possible, include some sort of incentive (or Stephenson's facilitator) for behavior change. This could be something specific, such as "free" or "low-cost" screenings to appeal to those who think the rich get better treatment than the poor, offering screenings at convenient times (especially evenings and weekends) for those who think getting the health care they need is too much trouble, providing free transportation from housing developments to clinics sites for those who believe transportation is a barrier to obtaining health care, and so on.

Specific concerns that differentiate the types also should be addressed. For example, The Empathizers are somewhat inclined to stay away from doctors because they may fear that doctors will tell them they are ill. Messages designed for them should stress the importance of screening for peace of mind or to set a positive example for family members. They likely will not be receptive to a message that reminds them that screenings find illnesses. It is important to identify and counter message dissonance as much as possible, especially for those individuals who will be difficult to motivate.

An awareness or education component is very important. The one knowledge question included in the telephone survey indicates that almost half of those surveyed do not know that African Americans are more likely than Caucasians to die from preventable or treatable diseases. African Americans are a bit more aware of the discrepancy than Caucasians, but close to one-third of the African Americans did not demonstrate an awareness of this fact. Also, symptoms and screening methods are likely not to be well known, especially among African Americans.

Another approach that can be effective with African Americans is modeling. If messages utilize black speech and culture and if they repeatedly show or applaud desired behavior, then the messages will have a cumulative effect. For example, if messages show over and over African American people going to get screenings, then it might motivate members of the target audience to follow suit. First, the individual will perceive the portrayed behavior. He or she will then judge the act of going for a screening as potentially useful to promote good health. The person will then get the screening and be rewarded with better health. This will lead to forming the habit of getting screenings on a regular basis. As previously discussed, modeling theory argues for long-term health care campaigns with as much media saturation as possible.

In utilizing the uses and gratifications model, attention should be paid to cognitive needs (ways that individuals acquire information, knowledge, and understanding). This involves how people process health information they obtain from doctors, family, friends, and the media. Affective needs, such as the desire for good health, come into play. Personal integrative needs involve reassurance that steps are being taken to assure better health for oneself or one's family. Social integrative needs are met through membership in support groups and social organizations. Finally, tension-release needs for escape and diversion, can be identified. Although it may be difficult to work these into a health campaign, letting people know that there is hope—in the form of relief of symptoms, cures, or management—can greatly relieve anxiety.

The diffusion model also should be used in campaign planning. It can be an effective way to formulate messages. First, messages should examine the relative advantage of participating in health care screenings. The relative advantage can be different for each of the types. For example, both The Equalizers and The Preventers are concerned about taking preventive actions that will save them money in the long run. The relative advantage for them could be saving money that might otherwise have to be spent on hospital bills and medications. On the other hand, The Empathizers are concerned about dignity and not being labeled or placed in a group. Screenings for them could promote the feeling of being included in an inclusive health care system.

Compatibility should be stressed in messages. Screenings should be viewed as part of an effective health care regiment rather than as a separate activity. The Adjusters, for example, do not believe that everyone has equal access to health care. For this type, access is viewed as being compatible with their ideal health care system. Also, as previously mentioned, those who want to save money will view screenings as being compatible with their goals and desire for preventive action.

As much as possible, health care messages should avoid complex explanations and plans of action. Keeping the message simple and the required action as easy as possible will be effective. This is especially important for those in every type who find getting health care too much trouble.

Trialability is extremely important for this type of health care campaign. Once people have gotten screenings, they may realize how quick and easy the process is. However, it is important that people are treated courteously and that discomfort be minimized. For example, long lines, emphasis on insurance, or physical pain inflicted during the screenings will not encourage people to form the habit of getting regular screenings. A pleasant experience, however, will result in more willingness to repeat the action.

Observability may be a bit difficult for this type of campaign, except that it likely will be beneficial to show a person being screened in promotional material. Showing a person who is relaxed and not in pain can help those people who try to avoid doctors overcome some of their fear. It is particularly important that African Americans be used in brochures or television commercials so that the message that screenings are only for white people will not be conveyed.

In this case, screenings are not really "new" or "innovative" techniques. Rather, making screenings available in non-traditional medical settings, i.e., churches or shopping centers, is the innovation. The goal should be to first introduce the innovation and then seek ways to "push" the adoption curve.

Early adopters should be encouraged to tell others in their network about the advantages of screening and to urge others to be screened. An "each one teach one" approach should be used if possible. Physicians should not be overlooked in the diffusion process. It is obvious from this study that physicians are the No. 1 interpersonal source of information for the vast majority of people. This is especially true of African Americans. Consequently, physicians need to be made aware of clinics and should be encouraged to refer patients to screen clinics for routine checkups. In Kansas City, for example, Dr. Jasper Fullard has a tremendous impact on clinic use because he encourages his diabetic patients to use the clinics as a less expensive alternative to office visits. Conversely, the clinic nurses make sure that people with positive test results for diabetes or high blood pressure are referred to doctors or clinics in their areas.

DEFINING COMMUNITIES

One requirement of communication may well be a shared environment that includes social, physical, and temporal space within a set of boundaries. Therefore, a campaign that targets inner-city African Americans needs to be aware of "communities" within these boundaries. Although it is still quite possible to locate communities with geographic boundaries (bounded by particular streets or zip code zones), being a member of a black community may be more a state of mind than a physical location. For example, as African Americans have become more affluent and moved into the middle and upper classes, they have moved from inner-city or rural areas into the suburbs. There is no longer a geographic connection, but there likely is an emotional and ethnic connection to a large and general black community. This may take the form of church membership or being active in social or political groups that are still primarily black.

For these reasons, it is important to identify institutions that are controlled by African Americans and that show concern for the problems African Americans face. Obviously, some of these can be located in a geographic area, such as neighborhood civic centers or youth centers. They should include black churches and clinics. On a larger scale, they can be social organizations, such as predominately black Mardi Gras krewes in Baton Rouge or groups like 100 Black Men in Kansas City. They should include medical support groups or health promotion groups, such as the Sickle Cell Anemia Foundation in Baton Rouge, the Black Health Care Coalition in St. Louis, and the diabetes support group in St. Louis.

Whatever communities are identified, it should be remembered that especially The Preventers and The Fixers believe that it is important for campaigns to originate at the local level. Even if the campaign originates at the state or national level, there should be a community component if at all possible. There must be a sense of ownership before the opinion leaders so important in diffusion and network theory can be utilized. Therefore, opinion leaders should be identified and consulted in planning the campaign.

Obviously, black churches and ministers are good places to start. There is generally an acceptance of black churches as having a role in promoting physical, as well as spiritual, health. But, support groups also are recognized as important, especially by The Adjusters and The Preventers.

PSYCHOGRAPHICS, LIFESTYLES, SUBCULTURES, SOCIAL RELATIONSHIPS

Psychographics and lifestyles are primarily marketing terms, and they should be considered in any health campaign. Aside from the collection of the Q data, this study did not devote much time to psychographics and lifestyles beyond an attempt to see if some groups are more health conscious than others. This took the form of asking for reported behavior changes (better diet, more exercise, etc.) and for current behavior patterns (smoking and drinking). Obviously, a much more detailed questionnaire could be designed to assess more specific eating and exercise habits, along with more emphasis on attitudes toward specific health habits or problems.

Subcultures also are given little attention in this particular survey, but the Q types are clues that there are at least two subcultures that must be kept in mind. The first is the poor, under-educated African American and the second is the affluent, educated African American. Although both groups may share some culture because of struggles against racial discrimination, they may view the world quite differently. For example, one group may see African Americans as victims of government and society, while the other group resists the "victim" image. Of course, subcultures also can have their own languages, modes of dress, and so on. These are important in that meanings attached to symbols can vary greatly from subculture to subculture. Any that might interfere with the communication process should be identified and countered if possible.

The multi-step flow theory and agenda setting model also have shown that discussions with friends, relatives, or acquaintances can be more important than the media in establishing opinions and attitudes. Although they are not ranked as highly as physicians, they are still important to a large segment of the subjects interviewed in the telephone survey. In fact, 30% of those surveyed listed family members or friends and acquaintances as their No. 1 interpersonal source of health information.

There are multiple ways to identify opinion leaders. It can be as simple as asking people to whom they turn for information and leadership. Content analysis of local media can determine who is most often quoted or used as expert sources. Relying heavily on ministers, educators, politicians, and presidents of various social organizations also is possible. Further, persons designated as opinion leaders are more exposed to radio, newspapers, and magazines, so a media use survey that includes demographics also can be useful in locating those who are likely to be most influential. There is evidence in the survey that a segment of the audience, i.e., The Empathizers, rely more on interpersonal communication than on the mass media for information. It is critical, therefore, that both physicians and community opinion leaders be drawn into this type of health care campaign.

MESSAGE DISPERSION STRATEGIES

There are multitudes of outlets for campaign messages, but the difficulty is in knowing which ones will be most effective. Almost 50% of the African Americans who participated in the telephone survey said they watch television more than 15 hours a week (25% watch more than 25 hours a week). The problem with using television is that although there can be heavy viewership, attention can be divided across a number of channels and programs. The social marketer must delve deeper into viewer habits to find which television shows are being watched (or at least during which time slots most African Americans are tuning in). This information also could be collected for each Q type.

Obviously, black media has been underutilized as an outlet for health care information. The focus groups for the American Newspaper Publishers Association's study of black newspapers revealed that many African Americans will welcome a health page in black newspapers. There are a few problems with using black media, newspapers in particular. Black newspapers often are not as professional-looking as mainstream newspapers. They lack the resources to take action photographs, to use spot color, or to have a team of reporters who can give the community thorough coverage. Furthermore, they may depend on cigarette and liquor company advertisements for survival. Consequently, they may not be viewed as the most credible of newspapers. Because credibility is crucial to health communication, the newspaper's credibility must be evaluated. However, 64% of the African Americans in the telephone survey said they subscribe to or regularly read a newspaper, and 57% said they read black newspapers. Campaign planners should realize that they would reach most of the reading African American audience through black newspapers (at least in areas where there are black newspapers). However, it is important to use mainstream newspapers, also, to increase the credibility of the message and to create awareness among as large a percentage of the total population as possible.

Although there is a statistically significant difference between the races in newspaper readership, there is no difference in the number of hours per week they listen to radio. Only about 11% of the African Americans surveyed by telephone said they did not listen to the radio. Furthermore, nearly 70% of the African Americans questioned said they listen to a radio station that programs primarily for blacks. Using black radio—through talk shows, newscasts, and public service announcements—to distribute health care messages is an effective means of communication.

Depending on the funds available, campaign planners should look at the feasibility of using direct mail, magazines (especially any that might be produced by local hospitals or health groups), newsletters, billboards, and pamphlets or brochures placed in physicians' offices, clinics, and hospitals as channels for the target messages. But, above all, attempts to influence through the mass media should coincide with interpersonal communication to increase the chances of success. Undoubtedly, the assistance of African American ministers, physicians, and educators should be enlisted along with the placement of media messages in both black and mainstream media.

Planners also should enlist the aid of the media to increase coverage of the black health care issue. Mainstream media often give little attention to stories that editors and reporters believe will appeal to a limited audience. Consequently, editors and reporters need to be made aware of the discrepancies in health between the races and encouraged to report on these problems. Agenda setting theory indicates that the media can be extremely important in bringing issues to the forefront.

COORDINATION WITH OTHER PROGRAMS

Because this campaign is theoretical, it is difficult to show how it might be coordinated with other programs. If this campaign were implemented, a review of hospital and clinic screening efforts, programs from groups such as The American Heart Association and the American Diabetes Society, and state Health Department programs should be undertaken to see what messages and networks have already been established. The next step is to determine whether there are areas of shared interest or financial support. Sometimes, testing data (surveys, focus groups, gathered statistics) can be obtained for use in the new campaign.

Above all, it is important to synchronize or harmonize messages (unless there is a deliberate need to counter some organization's or businesses' messages, i.e. cigarette company's messages, erroneous advertising, etc.) to avoid dissonance or the creation of unnecessary resistance.

TESTING

Social marketing principles dictate that thorough testing be done at every step of the campaign process. The amount and methods of testing may depend on both monetary restraints and personnel, but at the very least, messages should be tested as thoroughly as possible. One effective method of testing messages with small samples is to develop the messages and then have representatives from each of the Q types sort them as they previously sorted statements. This method not only would give an overall ranking of the messages, it would match messages to types.

In addition, messages should be tested for reading level, clarity, and impact. It is important to identify resistance points to the messages. Social marketers also are interested in message acceptability, believability, motivation, and conviction. A few in-depth, personal interviews or two or three focus groups can help in accessing these variables.

Once the messages have been disseminated, larger-scale telephone surveys or some type of panel design can test for recognition and recall of messages. Along with message recall, knowledge, attitude, and behavior measures also can be added.

The best effectiveness test is tracking of the number of screenings conducted. On-site evaluations also can be conducted. People who come for screenings can be asked a few simple questions, such as how they learned about the clinic and what most motivated them to come for a screening. This information can then be used to form new messages both to broaden the message appeal and to reinforce positive attitudes as they develop toward screening.

Also, barriers should be identified at every stage. Initial barriers may include lack of knowledge or misinformation about screenings. Later barriers could include inconvenient screening times, patient difficulty in reaching screening sites, long waiting times, sloppy screening procedures, and various negative attitudes that could surface about screenings in general. The purpose of identifying them, of course, is to launch "counter attacks" to overcome resistance points.

CONCLUSIONS

The ultimate goal of any health communications campaign should be convergence, moving people toward one point, to find a common focus. This involves trying to reach a mutual understanding. Several theories of communication and marketing strategies that can be used to achieve convergence have been discussed. They have been combined in a way to show that it is possible to target attitudes and behaviors of African Americans and attempt to move them toward the convergence of behaviors and attitude that can, in fact, produce better health.

This research indicates that African Americans and Caucasians share many attitudes so merely trying to divide the audience along racial lines is as inadequate as trying to divide them along demographic lines. Q methodology is critical in determining where attitudes overlap and where they diverge in the real world. For example, the analysis of the Q types indicate that middle class blacks and whites have more attitudes in common than upper income whites and low income blacks. Consequently, some health care campaigns can be reasonably affective for both African Americans and Caucasians if they have some demographic and psychographic factors in common. However, a campaign aimed at middle income whites will likely fail to change either attitudes or behaviors among low income blacks or high income whites. A national health campaign, therefore, must be designed to appeal to a minimum of three populations if it has as its goal behavior changes among the majority of the population (i.e., campaigns that have as goals reducing smoking or drinking or promoting safe sex).

The point is that instead of assuming that economic disadvantages doom segments of the population to poor health, attitudes that influence health behavior should be examined and possibly manipulated in ways to encourage all African Americans, especially those who are economically disadvantaged, to seek and find the health care they need.

This study has successfully demonstrated that there are attitudinal differences between African Americans and Caucasians that contribute to the discrepancies in health status between the two races. It also has shown that there are ways to attack and change these attitudes to increase African American participation in the American health care system. There are still many barriers to overcome, but at least efforts can and should be made to encourage full participation by both races.

Q Methodology Principles

Stephenson referred to the volume of discussion on a given topic as a "concourse." Brown listed six principles concerning measurement of the concourse:

1. The statements of a concourse, like particles in a liquid state, have no predetermined order or importance.
2. There is no standard Q sample for a concourse: Any suitably comprehensive sample is adequate for purposes of experimentation.
3. The measure of a person's subjective point of view can only be given by the person; it cannot be gained from the external 'objective' standpoint.
4. The forced-frequency Q-sort distribution is a theoretical expression of the law of error and not a statistical hypothesis for testing.
5. By the same token, there is no factor-analytic or related algorithm the mathematical and geometric formulations of which are valid across all problems—hence the value of the centroid method (the solution of which is indeterminate)and the problem-centeredness of theoretical rotation.
6. The fact that what statements mean can only be determined (by interpretation) after the factors are first found demonstrates that order precedes meaning. (In the scales of R methodology, by contrast, meanings precede order.) [1]

Stephenson characterized Q methodology as a set of philosophical, statistical, and psychometric ideas oriented to research on the individual.[2] In an article published in 1983, he wrote:

> Q sorts are probability distributions determined by feeling-state vectors, inseparably related to the defined psychological experience. . . . A

statement's positions are *developed* as a result of experiments in factor-analysis; and statements cannot be said "to have positions" before this experimentation. The statements form an ensemble and do not retain any individuality as such (the same statement has different meanings on different factors in the one factor-structure).[3]

Kerlinger said, "*Q technique* is a set of procedures used to implement Q methodology. It centers particularly in sorting decks of cards called *Q sorts* and in the correlations among the responses of different individuals to the *Q sorts*."[4]

Churchill, in his book, *Marketing Research Methodological Foundations*, describes the Q sort technique as a "general methodology for gathering data and processing the information collected. The task of the subjects in a Q sort analysis parallels that for the judgment sample in developing a Thurstone equal-appearing interval scale except (1) the subjects respond to each stimulus in terms of their attitudes toward it and not in terms of its degree of favorableness; (2) the subjects are instructed to place a specific number of statements in each category—that is, a distribution of responses is forced on the subject. Very often the specified distribution is normal or quasi-normal."[5] The subject does not merely agree or disagree with each statement, but actually ranks each statement in comparison with every other statement in the Q sample. Unlike R methodology, in which statements are ranked *independently*, Q methodology permits the rating of statements *interdependently*.

Brown said the first axiom of Q methodology is that it is the "subjective self" that is at the center of all meaning. This method is concerned with "states of mind" rather than observable states. Further, Brown points out that Q factors are indeterminant:

> We can never predict with certainty, particularly at the level of the single case, exactly how many factors will emerge, nor what their form and structure will be.[6]

There are eight steps involved in Q methodology, which can be described as "a set of techniques by which people can express their subjectivity—their thoughts, their feelings, their attitudes, their emotions, etc."[7] The steps are:

1. Selection of the Q sample—the stimulus items
2. Selection of the P sample—the subjects
3. Q sorting

4. Correlation of Q sorts
5. Factor analysis
6. Factor rotation
7. Compilation of weighted factor arrays
8. Interpretation of Q factors[8]

These steps as they relate to this study will be discussed below.

SELECTING THE Q SAMPLE

The procedure involves collecting a large number of self-referent (opinion) statements (which often begin "I think. . ." or "I believe. . ." or "In my opinion. . .") which are classified into categories or underlying structures. Stephenson often used either literature or face-to-face interviews to capture the statements. In this case literature sources were unlikely to yield African American opinion statements, and face-to-face interviews were too costly and time consuming. The alternative was four group discussions.

Nyamathi and Shuler provide a thorough discussion of the pros and cons of the focus group interview, which is "a qualitative research method for gathering information which, when performed in a permissive non-threatening group environment, allows the investigation of a multitude of perceptions on a defined area of interest."[9] They describe it as the "systematic study of the world of everyday experience."[10]

Patterson said the next step in the methodology "is to make use of Q sorting to model 'attitudes of mind' with respect to such opinions."[11] In Stephenson's view, there can be numerous opinions about a controversial issue, but only a few consonant and broad attitudes of mind, and still fewer belief-systems.[12] Once the statements are selected and the distribution decided, the next step is to select the subjects who will complete the sorts. As Patterson explains:

> Ordinarily in psychology and sociology one resorts to a sampling of populations of individuals, either on a random or a representative basis. In experimental psychology, however, much is learned in a scientific way by studying quite small numbers of persons, who are not randomly selected, but who are put into experimental and control groups, or in matched groups, etc. to answer set questions. Stephenson selects individuals in this manner, to represent different *interests* and the like as acceptable facts. He suggests how to measure public opinion, following the suggestions made in 1870 by G. Carslake Thompson, by representing different "interests" in experimental-type designs, called P sets or P samples.[13]

CALCULATION OF FACTORS

Following is a brief explanation of how the factors are calculated. The first factor chosen is the one along which the data are most "spread out," and will account for the maximum possible variation in the data. The second factor is selected so that it will account for the greatest possible amount of the remaining variance in the data. Additional factors are selected until the amount of unexplained variation remaining is below an acceptable limit.[14]

In addition to factor loadings, two other terms are important to the concept of factor analysis. The *communality* is the proportion of the person's variability that is explained by the factors. It is the sum of the squared loadings for the person across the factors.[15] Brown points out that communality (h^2) is important because during rotation the factor loadings change although the sum of the squared factor loadings should still equal the original value of h^2 no matter how changed the loadings may be.[16] For each factor, the *eigenvalue* is the sum of the squared factor loadings for that factor.[17] The percentage of total variance accounted for by each factor is equal to the eigenvalue divided by the number of persons in the P sample.[18] For this study, factors with an eigenvalue of 1 or higher are considered significant.

Once the factors have been determined, it is possible to see an array of statements with z scores to show which statements were placed similarly by the subjects who make up the factor. Some statements can be consensus statements, that is nearly everyone, regardless of the factors, tended to agree or disagree with the statement. For example, as the following table shows, nearly everyone completing the Q sort agreed that federal policies prohibiting discrimination should be enforced. Likewise, no one sorting the statements indicated they would be more likely to use an emergency room than a private doctor.

TABLE 35
CONSENSUS STATEMENTS

Statements	Average Z-Score
23. Federal policies prohibiting discrimination in health service delivery should be enforced.	.95
15. If you have an important message about health-care, put it on television.	.44
25. Any successful health campaign that could change behaviors would originate in my community rather than at the state, national level.	.42
11. In health care promotions and advertising, white faces bringing bad news to blacks will not work.	-.20
10. Getting the health care I need is usually too much trouble.	-.97
16. If I need medical care, I will most likely go to a hospital emergency room rather than to a private physician.	-1.19

Author's Note:

For additional information about the survey instruments, list of Q sort statements, a summary of Q subject backgrounds, and a summary of the telephone survey results, see the dissertation on which this book is based: *Directing Health Messages Toward African Americans: Attitudes Toward Health Care and the Mass Media*, UMI Microform #9620235.

NOTES

1. Steven R. Brown, *Political Subjectivity: Applications of Q Methodology in Political Science*, (New Haven: Yale University, 1980), 74-75.

2. William Stephenson, *The Study of Behavior*, (Chicago: University of Chicago Press, 1953) cited in Fred N. Kerlinger, *Foundations of Behavioral Research*, 2d., (New York: Holt, Rinehart and Winston, Inc., 1973, 582.

3. William Stephenson, "Quantum Theory and Q-methodology: Fictionalistic and Probabilistic Theories Conjoined," *The Psychological-Record*, 33 (Spring 1983), 215.

4. Fred N. Kerlinger, *Foundations of Behavioral Research*, 2d., (New York: Holt, Rinehart and Winston, Inc., 1973, 582.

5. Churchill, 336.

6. Brown, 73.

7. Keith P. Sanders, "Q Methodology—An Overview," Handout for Advanced Research Methods class, University of Missouri, Winter, 1986, 1.

8. Ibid.

9. Adline Nyamathi and Pam Shuler, "Focus Group Interview: A Research Technique for Informed Nursing Practice," *Journal of Advanced Nursing*, 15, (1990), 1282.

10. Ibid.

11. Patterson, 33.

12. William Stephenson, "Definition of Opinion, Attitude and Belief," *The Psychological- Record*, April 1965, 281-288.

13. Patterson, 35.

14. Ronald M. Weiers, *Marketing Research*, 2d. ed., (Englewood Cliffs, N.J.: Prentice Hall, 1988), 503.

15. Ibid., 505.

16. Brown, 223-224.

17. Ibid.

18. Ibid., 40.

Bibliography

A. BOOKS

Assael, H. *Consumer Behavior and Marketing Action*. 2d. ed., Boston: Kent Publishers, 1984.

Atkin, Charles and Elaine Bratic Arkin. "Issues and Initiatives in Communicating Health Information to the Public, " in *Mass Communication and Public Health: Complexities and Conflicts*, edited by Charles Atkin and Lawrence Wallack. Newbury Park, CA: Sage Publications, Inc., 1990.

———— and Lawrence Wallack, eds. *Mass Communication and Public Health: Complexities and Conflicts*. Newbury Park, CA: Sage Publications, Inc., 1990.

Backer, Thomas E. and Ginna Marston. "Partnership for a Drug-Free America: An Experiment in Social Marketing," in *Organizational Aspects of Health Communication Campaigns: What Works?*, edited by Thomas E. Backer and Everett M. Rogers. Newbury Park, CA: Sage Publications, Inc., 1993.

———— and Everett M. Rogers, eds. *Organizational Aspects of Health Communication Campaigns: What Works?* Newbury Park, CA: Sage Publications, Inc., 1993.

Becker, Lee B., Idowa A. Sobowale; Robin E. Cobbey; and Chaim H. Eyal. "Debates' Effects on Voters' Understanding of Candidates and Issues," *The Presidential Debates: Media, Electoral, and Policy Perspectives*. Edited by George F. Bishop, Robert G. Meadow, and Marilyn Jackson-Beeck. New York: Praeger, 1978.

Berelson, B. and G. Steiner. *Human Behavior*. New York: Harcourt and Brace, 1964.

Brown, Steven R. *Political Subjectivity: Applications of Q Methodology in Political Science*. New Haven: Yale University, 1980.

Churchill Jr., Gilbert A. *Marketing Research Methodological Foundations*, 4th ed., Chicago: The Dryden Press, 1987.

Cohen, Bernard. *The Press and Foreign Policy*. Princeton, NJ: Princeton University Press, 1963.

Davison, W. Phillips , James Boylan, and Frederick T.C. Yu. *Mass Media Systems & Effects*. 2d ed., New York: CBS College Publishing, 1982.

DeFleur, Melvin L. and Sandra Ball-Rokeach. *Theories of Mass Communication.* 5th ed., White Plains, NY: Longman Inc., 1989.

———. *Theories of Mass Communication.* New York: David McKay Company, Inc., 1966.

Deutscher, I. *Words and Deeds: Social Science and Social Policy.* Reprinted from *Social Problems,* 13 (1966) 233-254, in *The Sociologist as Detective,* edited by W. Saunders. New York: Praeger Publishers, 1976.

Devine, Patricia G. and Edward R. Hirt. "Message Strategies for Information Campaigns: A Social-Psychological Analysis," in *Information Campaigns: Balancing Social Values and Social Change,* edited by Charles T. Salmon. Newbury Park, CA: Sage Publications, Inc., 1989.

Festinger, Leon . "The Theory of Cognitive Dissonance." Chap. in *The Science of Human Communication.* New York: Basic Books, Inc., 1963.

Finnegan, Jr., John R., Neil Bracht, and K. Viswanath, "Community Power and Leadership Analysis in Lifestyle Campaigns," in *Information Campaigns: Balancing Social Values and Social Change,* edited by Charles T. Salmon. Newbury Park, CA: Sage Publications, Inc., 1989.

Fitzpatrick, J. *Puerto Rican Americans: The Meaning of Migration to the Mainland.* Englewood Cliffs, N.J.: Prentice-Hall, 1971.

Flay, Brian R. and Dee Burton. "Effective Mass Communication Strategies for Health Campaigns." In *Mass Communication and Public Health: Complexities and Conflicts,* edited by Charles Atkin and Lawrence Wallack. Newbury Park, CA: Sage Publications, Inc., 1990.

Flora, June A., Darius Jatilus, Chris Jackson, and Stephen P. Fortmann. "The Stanford Five-City Heart Disease Prevention Project," in *Organizational Aspects of Health Communication Campaigns: What Works?,* edited by Thomas E. Backer and Everett M. Rogers. Newbury Park, CA: Sage Publications, Inc., 1993.

Gandy, Oscar. *Beyond Agenda Setting: Information Subsidies and Public Policies.* Norwood, N.J.: Ablex Publishing Company, 1982.

Grunig, James E. "Publics, Audiences and Market Segments: Segmentation Principles for Campaigns," in *Information Campaigns: Balancing Social Values and Social Change,* edited by Charles T. Salmon. Newbury Park, CA: Sage Publications, Inc., 1989.

Hancock, Alan. *Mass Communication.* New York: Longman Group Limited, 1970.

Hornik, Robert. "The Knowledge-Behavior Gap in Public Information Campaigns: A Development Communication View," in *Information Campaigns: Balancing Social Values and Social Change,* edited by Charles T. Salmon. Newbury Park, CA: Sage Publications, Inc., 1989.

Katz, Elihu, Jay G. Blumler, and Michael Gurevitch. "Uses of Mass Communication by the Individual," *Mass Communication Research.* eds. W. Phillips Davison and Frederick T.C. Yu, New York: Praeger, 1974.

———, and Paul Lazarsfeld. *Personal Influence: The Part Played by People in the Flow of Mass Communications.* Glencoe, IL: The Free Press, 1955.

Kerlinger, Fred N. *Foundations of Behavioral Research.* 2d. ed., New York: Holt, Rinehart and Winston, Inc., 1973.

Kirkpatrick, C.A. *Advertising, Mass Communication in Marketing.* Boston: Houghton Mifflin Co., 1964.

Klapper, Joseph T. *The Effects of the Mass Media.* Glencoe, Ill.: The Free Press of Glencoe, 1960.

————. *The Effects of Mass Communication.* Glencoe, Illinois: The Free Press, 1960.

Lazarsfeld, Paul, Bernard Berelson, and Hazel Gaudet. *The People's Choice.* New York: Columbia University Press, 1940.

Lowery, Shearon and Melvin L. DeFleur. *Milestones in Mass Communication Research: Media Effects.* White Plains, NY: Longman Inc., 1983.

Manoff, Richard K. *Social Marketing: New Imperative for Public Health.* New York: Praeger Publishers, 1985.

McQuail, Denis, Jay G. Blumler, and J. Brown, "The Television Audience: A Revised Perspective," in D. McQuail (ed.), *Sociology of Mass Communication.* Harmondsworth, England: Penguin, 1972.

Meyer, Philip. "News Media Responsiveness to Public Health," in *Mass Communication and Public Health: Complexities and Conflicts,* edited by Charles Atkin and Lawrence Wallack. Newbury Park, CA: Sage Publications, Inc., 1990.

Pentz, Mary Ann and Thomas W. Valente, "Project Star: A Substance Abuse Prevention Campaign in Kansas City," in *Organizational Aspects of Health Communication Campaigns: What Works?,* edited by Thomas E. Backer and Everett M. Rogers. Newbury Park, CA: Sage Publications, Inc., 1993.

Quera, Leon. *Advertising Campaigns: Formulation and Tactics.* 2d ed., Columbus, Ohio: Grid Inc., 1977.

Reissman F. ed. *Mental Health of the Poor.* New York: The Free Press, 1964.

Rogers, Everett M. and J.D. Storey. "Communication Campaigns," in *Handbook of Communication Science,* edited by C.R. Berger and S.H. Chaffee. Newbury Park, CA: Sage Publications, Inc., 1988.

————. and F. Floyd Shoemaker. *Communication of Innovations.* New York: The Free Press, 1971.

————. *Diffusion of Innovations.* 3d ed. New York: The Free Press, Div. Macmillan Publishing Co., Inc., 1983.

———— and D. Lawrence Kincaid, *Communication Networks: Toward a New Paradigm for Research,* (New York: The Free Press, 1981), 62.

Salmon, Charles T. "Campaigns for Social 'Improvement': An Overview of Values, Rationales, and Impacts," in *Information Campaigns: Balancing Social Values and Social Change,* edited by Charles T. Salmon. Newbury Park, CA: Sage Publications, Inc., 1989.

Stephenson, William. *The Play Theory of Mass Communication.* Chicago: University of Chicago Press, 1967.

————. Foreword to *Political Subjectivity: Applications of Q Methodology in Political Science* by Steven R. Brown. New Haven: Yale University, 1980.

————. *The Study of Behavior.* Chicago: University of Chicago Press, 1953.

Tichenor, Phillip .J., G.A. Donohue, and C.N. Olien. *Community Conflict and the Press.* Beverly Hills, CA: Sage, 1980.

————. *Community Conflict and the Press.* Beverly Hills, Ca.: Sage, 1980.

Weiers, Ronald M. *Marketing Research.* 2d. ed., Englewood Cliffs, N.J.: Prentice Hall, 1988.

Wright, John S. and Daniel S. Warner. *Advertising.* New York: McGraw-Hill Book Co., 1966.

B. DISSERTATIONS

Olins, Robert Abbot. "A Model Study of an Advertising Campaign." Ph.D. diss., University of Missouri, 1971.

Patterson, Joye. "Attitudes About Science: A Dissection." Ph.D. diss., University of Missouri, 1966.

Shipley, Linda Mahoney. "A Q-Methodology Study of Information and Opinion-Seeking." M.A. thesis., University of Missouri, 1969.

C. NEWSPAPERS/WIRE SERVICE

Adler, Eric . "Disease: Another Black Burden." *The Kansas City Star*, 24 July 1991, 1 (A).

Adler, Eric. "A Race at Risk." *The Kansas City Star*, 24 July 1991, A (8).

The Associated Press. "Report Attests to Success of Calif. Anti-Smoking Campaign." *The Daily Advocate*, 21 March 1994, 12 (A).

AP Online. "Medicare No Longer a Sacred Cow," Prodigy Services Co., 26 June 1997 and "Medicare Changes May Fight Waste," Prodigy Services Co., 27 June 1997.

AP Online. "Shift to Managed Care is Inevitable," Prodigy Services Co., 2 July 1997.

Lagnado, Lucette . "When Racial Sensitivities Clash with Research." *The Wall Street Journal,* 25 June 1997 B(1).

D. PERIODICALS

Abad, Vicente, Juan Ramos and Elizabeth Boyce, "A Model for Delivery of Mental Health Services to Spanish-Speaking Minorities." *American Journal of Orthopsychiatry*, 44 (4), (July 1974), 584-595.

Ajzen, I. and M. Fishbein. "Attitude-Behavior Relations: A Theoretical Analysis and Review of Empirical Research." *Psychological Bulletin,* 84, (1977), 888-918.

Anderson, Robert M., W.H. Herman, J.M. Davis, R.P. Freedman, M.M. Funnell, and H.W. Neighbors. "Barriers to Improving Diabetes Care for Blacks." *Diabetes Care*, Vol. 14, No. 7, (July 1991): 605-609.

Berkanovic, E. and C. Telesky. "Mexican-American, Black-American and White-American Differences in Reporting Illnesses, Disability and Physician Visits for Illnesses." *Social Science in Medicine*, 20, (1985): 567-577.

Blendon, Robert J., L.H. Aiken, H.E. Freeman, and C.R. Corey. "Access to Medical Care for Black and White Americans A Matter of Continuing Concern." *Journal of the American Medical Association*, Vol. 261, No. 2, (1989): 278-281.

Block, Carl E. "Communicating with the Urban Poor: an Exploratory Inquiry." *Journalism Quarterly*, (Spring, 1970): 3-11.

Boring, Catherine C., Teresa S. Squires and Clark W. Heath, Jr. "Cancer Statistics for African Americans." *CA—A Cancer Journal for Clinicians*, 41, (May/June 1991): 7-17.

Braveman, Paula, G. Oliva, M.G. Miller, V.M. Schaaf, and R. Reiter. "Women and Medicine: Women Without Health Insurance Links Between Access, Poverty, Ethnicity, and Health." *Western Journal of Medicine*, December (1988): 708-711.

Brownson, Ross C., James R. Davis, and Jian C. Chang. "Racial Differences in Cancer Mortality in Missouri." *Missouri Medicine*, (May, 1990): 291-294.

Cox, Donald F. "Clues for Advertising Strategists II." *Harvard Business Review*, 39(6), (1961): 160-182.

Cutlip, Scott M. "Third of Newspapers' Content PR Inspired." *Editor & Publisher*, (May 26, 1962).

Diehr, P. , D.P. Martin, K.F. Price et al., "Use of Ambulatory Care Services in Three Provider Plans." *American Journal of Public Health, 74, (*1984): 47-51.

Dignan, Mark, R. Michielutte, P. Shapr, J. Bahnson, L.Young, and P. Beal. "The Role of Focus Groups in Health Education for Cervical Cancer Among Minority Women." *Journal of Community Health*, 15, (December 1990): 369-375.

Doll, R. and R. Peto. "The Causes of Cancer. Quantitative Estimates of Avoidable Risks of Cancer in the United States Today." *Journal of National Cancer Institute*, 66, (1981): 1191-1308.

Egbert, L.D and I.L. Rothman, "Relation Between Race and Economic Status of Patients and Who Performs Their Surgery." *New England Journal of Medicine*, 297, (1977), 90- 91.

Gillum, R.F. "Coronary Heart Disease in Black Populations I: Mortality and Morbidity." *American Heart Journal.* 104, (1982): 839-851.

Gross, S.J. and C. Niman. "Attitude Behavior Consistency: A Review." *Public Opinion Quarterly*, 39, (1975), 358-368.

Gylys, J. and B. Gylys. "Cultural Influences and the Medical Behavior of Low Income Groups." *Journal of the National Medical Association*, 66, (1974): 310-313.

Hale, Christiane B., and Charlotte M. Druschel. "Infant Mortality Among Moderately Low Birth Weight Infants in Alabama, 1980 to 1983." *Pediatrics*, Vol. 84 No. 2, (August 1989): 285-289.

Haywood, L. Julian"Hypertension in Minority Populations," *The American Journal of Medicine*, 88 (suppl 3B), (March 12, 1990), 17s-20s.

Hopper, S. "Diabetes as a Stigmatized Condition: the Case of Low-Income Patients in the United States." *Social Science Medicine*, 15B, (1981): 11-19.

Kahn, Katherine L., Marjorie L. Pearson, Ellen R. Harrison, Katherine A. Desmond, William H. Rogers, Lisa V. Rubenstein, Robert H. Brook, and Emmett B. Keeler. "Health Care for Black and Poor Hospitalized Medicare Patients." *Journal of the American Medical Association*, Vol. 271 No. 15, (April 20, 1994): 1169-1174.

Katz, Elihu. "The Two-Step Flow of Communication: An Up-To-Date Report on an Hypothesis." *Public Opinion Quarterly* XXI (1957): 61-78.

Katz, Elihu, Michael Gurevitch, and Hadassah Haas, "On the Uses of the Mass Media for Important Things," *American Sociological Review*, 38, (1973): 164-181.

Keil, J.E., D.E. Saunders, D.T. Lackland, et al., "Acute Myocardial Infarction: Period Prevalence, Case Fatality and Comparison of Black and White Cases in Urban and Rural Areas of South Carolina." *America Heart Journal*, 109, (1985): 776-784.

Kenton, Edgar J. "Access to Neurological Care for Minorities." *Archives of Neurology*, 48, (May 1991): 480-483.

Knafl, K. and M. Howard, "Interpreting and Reporting Qualitative Research." *Research in Nursing and Health*, 7, 17-24.

Krugman, Herbert E. "The Impact of Television Advertising." *Public Opinion Quarterly*. 29, (1965): 349-356.

LaPiere, R.T. "Attitude vs. Action." *Social Forces*, 13 (1934): 230-237.

Lefebvre, R.C. and J.A. Flora, "Social Marketing and Public Health Interventions." *Health Education* Quarterly, 15, (1988), 299-315.

Maynard, L.D. Fisher, E.R. Passamani et al., "Blacks in the Coronary Artery Surgery Study." *Circulation*, 74, (1986:) 64-71.

McCombs, Maxwell E. and Donald L. Shaw. "Structuring the 'Unseen Environment.'" *Journal of Communication*, 26(2), (Spring, 1976): 18-22.

Menzel, Herbert and Elihu Katz. "Social Relations and Innovation in the Medical Profession: The Epidemiology of a New Drug." *Public Opinion Quarterly* XIX (Winter, 1955- 56), 338-352.

Mosher, J.F. and L.M. Wallack. "Proposed Reforms in the Regulation of Alcoholic Beverage Advertising." *Contemporary Drug Problem*, 8 (1979), 87-106.

Noelle-Neumann, E. "Return to the Concept of Powerful Mass Media." *Studies of Broadcasting*, (1973): 66-112.

Nyamathi, Adline and Pam Shuler. "Focus Group Interview: A Research Technique for Informed Nursing Practice," *Journal of Advanced Nursing*, 15, (1990), 1281-1288.

Olien, Clarice N., George A. Donohue, and Phillip Tichenor, "Media and Stages of Social Conflict." *Journalism Monographs*, 90, (November 1984): 1-31.

Petchers, Marcia K. and Sharon E. Milligan. "Access to Health Care in a Black Urban Elderly Populations." *Gerontologist*, Vol. 28 No. 2, (April 1988): 213-217.

Peterson, Eric D., Steven M. Wright, Jennifer Daley, George E. Thibault. "Racial Variation in Cardiac Procedure Use and Survival Following Acute Myocardial Infarction in the Department of Veterans Affairs." *Journal of the American Medical Association*, Vol. 271 No. 15, (April 20, 1994): 1175-1180.

Scupholme, Anne, Euan G. Robertson, and A. Susan Kamons. "Barriers to Prenatal Care in a Multiethnic, Urban Sample." *Journal of Nurse-Midwifery*, Vol. 36 No. 2, (March/April, 1991): 111-116.

Sharma, Arun. "The Persuasive Effect of Salesperson Credibility: Conceptual and Empirical Examination." *Journal of Personal Selling & Sales Managements*, 10 (Fall 1990), 71-80.

Shoemaker, P. "Deviance of Political Groups and Media Treatment." *Journalism Quarterly* 61 (1984): 66-75.

Sidel, Victor W. "The Health of Poor and Minority People in the Inner City." *New York State Journal of Medicine*, Vol. 91 No. 5, (May 1991), 180-182.

Smith, Kim. "Newspaper Coverage and Public Concern about Community Issues: A Time-Series Analysis." *Journalism Monographs*, 101 (February 1987): 1-32.

Stephenson, William. "Definition of Opinion, Attitude and Belief." *The Psychological- Record*, (April 1965): 281-288.

————. "Quantum Theory and Q-methodology: Fictionalistic and Probabilistic Theories Conjoined." *The Psychological-Record*, 33 (Spring 1983), 213-230.

Stern, M.P. "Results of a Two-Year Health Education Campaign on Dietary Behavior." *Circulation*, 54, (1976): 826-833.

Strogatz, David S. "Use of Medical Care for Chest Pain: Differences between Blacks and Whites." *American Journal of Public Health*, Vol. 80 No. 3, (March 1990): 290-294.

Tichenor, Phillip J., G.A. Donohue, and C.N. Olien. "Mass Media Flow and the Differential Growth of Knowledge." *Public Opinion Quarterly*, 34, (1970): 159-170.

Troldahl, Verling. "A Field Test of a Modified 'Two-Step Flow of Communication' Model." *Public Opinion Quarterly* XXX (Winter, 1966-67), 609-623.

VanSon, A.R. "Crossing Cultural and Economic Boundaries." In *Diabetes and Patient Education: A Daily Nursing Challenge* (New York: Appleton-Century-Crofts, 1981), 160-177.

Wallack, Lawrence M. "Mass Media Campaigns: The Odds Against Finding Behavior Change." *Health Education Quarterly* 8(3), (Fall, 1981): 209-257.

Weaver, David and Swanzy Nimley Elliott. "Who Sets the Agenda for the Media? A Study of Local Agenda Building." *Journalism Quarterly*, 62 (Spring 1985): 87-94.

Weisse, A.B. , P.D. Abiuso, and I.S. Thind. "Acute Myocardial Infarction in Newark, NJ," *Archives of Internal Medicine*, 137, 1977, 1402-1405.

Weissman, Joel S., R. Stern, S.L. Fielding, and A.M. Epstein. "Delayed Access to Health Care: Risk Factors, Reasons, and Consequences." *Annals of Internal Medicine*, Vol. 114 No. 4, (Feb. 15, 1991): 325-331.

White-Means, Shelly I. and Michael C. Thornton. "Nonemergency Visits to Hospital Emergency Rooms: A Comparison of Blacks and Whites." *The Milbank Quarterly*, Vol 67, No. 1, (1989): 35-57.

Wicker, A.W. "Attitudes Versus Actions: The Relationship of Verbal and Overt Behavioral Responses to Attitude Objects." *Journal of Social Issues*, 45 (1969), 65.

Wiebe, G.D. "Merchandising Commodities and Citizenship on Television." *Public Opinion Quarterly*, XXV (1951): 679-691.

Wilde, Gerald J.S. "Effects of Mass Media Communications on Health and Safety Habits: An Overview of Issues and Evidence." *Addiction* 88 (1993): 986-987.

Yergan, J., "Relationship Between Patient Race and the Intensity of Hospital Services." *Medical Care*, 25, (1987): 592-603.

E. PUBLIC DOCUMENTS AND REPORTS

Access to Health Care in the United States: Results of a 1986 Survey—Special Report No. 2. [Princeton, NJ]: Robert Wood Johnson Foundation, 1987.

American Diabetes Association. *Diabetes: An Equal Opportunity Disease,* [Alexandria, VA]: Diabetes Information Service Center, 1989.

Butler, P.A. "Too Poor to Be Sick: Access to Medical Care for the Uninsured." *American Public Health Association.* [Washington, D.C.]: 1988.

Council Report., *Black-White Disparities in Health Care,* [Chicago, IL]: Council on Ethical and Judicial Affairs, American Medical Association,, 1989.

Erdman, K. and S. Wolfe. *Poor Health Care for Poor Americans: A Ranking of State Medicaid Programs.* [Washington D.C.]: Public Citizen Health Research Group, 1987.

Health Status of the Disadvantaged—Chartbook 1986. United States. U.S. Department of Health and Human Services (DHHS) Publication No. HRS-P-DV86-2. [Washington, D.C.]: Health Resources and Services Administration, 1986.

Henderson, M.J. and D.D. Savage. "Prevalence and Incidence of Ischemic Heart Disease in United States' Black and White Populations." *Report of the Secretary's Task Force on Black and Minority Health IV Cardiovascular and Cerebrovascular Disease.* [Washington, D.C.]: Government Printing Office, (1986): 620-638.

Missouri Department of Health, State Center for Health Statistics. *Missouri Vital Statistics 1988.* [Jefferson City]: Missouri Department of Health, Division of Health Resources, State Center for Health Statistics, 1989.

National Center for Health Statistics. *Health, United States, 1987,* DHHS Publication (PHS) 88-1232. [Washington, D.C.]: Department of Health and Human Services, 1987.

National Center for Health Statistics, Bureau of Census. *Persons With and Without a Regular Source of Medical Care.* [Washington, D.C.]: Bureau of Census, Series 10, No. 151, 1985.

National Diabetes Data Group. *Diabetes in America.* [Bethesda, MD]: Department of Health and Human Services, NIH publication No. 85-1468, 1985.

National Center for Health Statistics. *Health United States 1984,* US DHHS Publication No. (PHS)85-1232. [Hyattsville, Md.]: National Center for Health Statistics, 1984.

Public Health Service Task Force on Women's Issues. *Women's Health Report,* [Washington, D.C.]: Department of Public Health, 100, 1985, 73-105.

Ries, L.A.G., B.F. Hankey, B.K. Edwards. *Cancer Statistics Review 1973-1988,.* NIH Publication No 91-2789, [Bethesda, MD]: National Cancer Institute, 1991.

Robert Wood Johnson Foundation Special Report. *Access to Health Care in the United States: Results of a 1986 Survey,* [Princeton, NJ]: Robert Wood Johnson Foundation, 1987.

U.S. Centers for Disease Control. Atlanta, Ga.: 1992.

U.S. Department of Commerce, Bureau of Census. *Current Population Survey,* [Washington, D.C.]: U.S. Department of Commerce, Bureau of Census, 1987.

U.S. Department of Health, Education and Welfare. *Health Status of Minorities and Low- Income Groups,* U.S. Department of Health, Education and Welfare (DHEW) publication No. HRA 790627. [Washington, D.C.]: U.S. Department of Health, Education and Welfare, Health Resources Administration, 1978.

U.S. Department of Health and Human Services. National Center for Health Statistics. Vital Statistics of the United States, 1979: *Mortality.* [Washington, D.C.]: U.S. Department of Health and Human Services Publication (PHS)84-1101 Public Health Service, 2 pt A, 1984.

U.S. Department of Health and Human Services. *Report of the Secretary's Task Force on Black Minority Health, VI: Infant Mortality and Low Birthweight.* [Washington, DC]: U.S. Department of Health and Human Services, 1986.

U.S. Department of Health and Human Services. *Report of the Secretary's Task Force on Black & Minority Health, VII, Chemical Dependency and Diabetes.* [Washington, D.C.]: U.S. Department of Health and Human Services, 1985.

U.S. Department of Health and Human Services. *Report of the Secretary's Task Force on Black & Minority Health. Volume III: Cancer.* [Washington D.C.]: U.S. Government Printing Office, DHHS Publication No. 86-621-605, 1986.

U.S. Public Health Service. *Cancer Among Blacks and Other Minorities: Statistical Profiles.* [Bethesda, MD]: U.S. Department of Health and Human Services, Public Health Service, National Cancer Institute, NIH Publication No. 86-2785, 1986.

U.S. Public Health Service. *1987 Annual Cancer Statistics Review Including Cancer Trends: 1950-1985.* [Bethesda, MD]: U.S. Department of Health and Human Services, Public Health Service, National Cancer Institute, NIH Publication No. 88-2789, 1988.

F. UNPUBLISHED DOCUMENTS AND PAPERS

Atkin, Charles K., Gina M. Garramone, and Ronald Anderson. *Formative Evaluation Research in Health Campaign Planning: The Case of Drunk Driving Prevention.*" Paper presented as part of the annual conference of International Communication Association, Health Communication Division, Chicago, May 1986.

Brenner, Donald J. "Beyond Diffusion: Network Analysis and Q." Paper presented at the second annual Conference on the Scientific Study of Subjectivity, Columbia, Mo., July, 1986.

Brown, William J. *Effects of an AIDS Prevention Campaign on Attitudes, Beliefs, and Communication Behavior.* Paper presented as part of the Health Communication Division of the 41st Annual Conference of the International Communication Association, Chicago, IL, 25 May 1991.

Hertog, James, John R. Finnegan Jr., K. Viswanath, Brenda Rooney, Judy Baxter, Patricia Elmer, Karen Graves, Rebecca Mullis, Phyllis Pirie, John Potter, and Leslie Trenkner. *Formative Analysis for Community-Based Health Campaigns: Experiences of the Cancer and Dietary Intervention Project.* Paper presented as part of the Health Communication Division of the 41st Annual Conference of the International Communication Association, Chicago, 25 May 1991.

Sanders, Keith P. "On Interpretation of Q Factors." Handout for Advanced Research Methods class, November 1972.

————. "Q Methodology—An Overview." Handout for Advanced Research Methods class, University of Missouri, Winter, 1986.

Stephenson, William. "The Vergent Report, April 1, 1967 - June 30, 1971." Western Historical Manuscript Collections, Ellis Library, University of Missouri, Columbia.

Sylvester, Judith. "Media Research Bureau Black Newspaper Readership Report," Sears Foundation/National Newspaper Publishers Association Report, University of Missouri: June 24, 1993.

Viswanath, K., John R. Finnegan Jr., Peter Hannan, and Russell V. Luepker. *Health and Knowledge Gaps: Some Lessons from the Minnesota Heart Health Program.* Paper presented as part of the annual conference of the International Communication Association, Chicago, IL, 23-27 May 1991.

Index